Does smoking really destroy the vitamin C in my body?

Do those body-building protein supplements really work?

What can I eat to help me get more iron?

What's the big deal about beta-carotene?

This is the book that answers your questions about vitamins . . . from A to Zinc. With a guide to vitamins and up-to-date information about your nutritional needs, it's the guide that provides the facts about vitamins—at your fingertips.

THE COMPLETE VITAMIN BOOK

THE COMPLETE VITAMIN BOOK

CARL LOWE

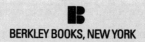

BERKLEY BOOKS, NEW YORK

THE COMPLETE VITAMIN BOOK

A Berkley Book / published by arrangement with the author

PRINTING HISTORY
Berkley edition / September 1994

All rights reserved.
Copyright © 1994 by Carl Lowe.
This book may not be reproduced in whole
or in part, by mimeograph or any other means,
without permission. For information address:
The Berkley Publishing Group,
200 Madison Avenue, New York, New York 10016.

ISBN: 0-425-14365-1

BERKLEY®
Berkley Books are published by The Berkley Publishing Group,
200 Madison Avenue, New York, New York 10016.
BERKLEY and the "B" design
are trademarks belonging to the Berkley Publishing Corporation.

PRINTED IN THE UNITED STATES OF AMERICA

10 9 8 7 6 5 4 3 2 1

Contents

THE COMPLETE VITAMIN BOOK

INTRODUCTION

Vitamins prove the old saying that good things come in small packages. If you took a chemically purified formula containing the total minimal daily amount of the known vitamins you need to survive and put them in a teaspoon, you would still have more than two-thirds of the spoon left over to fill with other nutrients. We only need microscopic amounts of vitamins to live, but those microscopic amounts make a big difference in the quality of our lives.

Most vitamins act as coenzymes in the human body. That means that they are assistants: They help enzymes do their jobs speedily and properly. Enzymes are catalysts that make the life processes work. They are inextricably involved in the body's absorption of food from the digestive tract; the movement of oxygen from our lungs to each cell; the creation of replacement parts for every section of our bodies including blood cells, bone, teeth, skin, and hormones; the protection of cells from disease-causing microbes; and the transmission of nerve signals. In other words, enzymes and coenzymes are necessary for everything from the reproduction of the skin cells on the back of your hand to the sexual reproduction of our species.

Chemical Protection

Beyond vitamins' basic tasks that keep our metabolic machinery running smoothly, researchers have found that these nutrients have protective functions as well. One of the most notable is their roles as antioxidants. In our day-to-day existence, our bodies ingest and produce substances known as oxidants that attack our cells and organs. Scientists now believe that oxidants play a major part in causing aging, cancer, and heart disease. The latest studies seem to confirm that vitamins, in conjunction with the body's other antioxidants, can defuse the destructive power of oxidants and preserve our health and well-being.

Discoveries such as these lead to controversy. If vitamins at minimal amounts keep us alive, some researchers ask, can larger amounts of these nutrients do more? Can megadoses of these micronutrients endow us with better health and longer and more productive lives? Beyond that, can we get all the vitamins we need from food or are vitamin pills always necessary for an optimal intake of vitamins?

These questions have led to a battle of the nutrition experts. On one side stand the traditionalists who insist on sticking to the "balanced diet" ethos. They believe that eating a wide variety of foods will supply all your necessary nutrients; that extra vitamins in supplements are at best useless and at worst dangerous because they may throw your nutritional balance out of whack; and that the research demonstrating the benefits of extra vitamins draw mistaken conclusions.

On the other side stands a growing band of scientists who point to a long list of studies showing benefits to people who take higher vitamin doses. They believe supplemental vitamins are responsible for drops in the rate of birth defects and to groups of people that live longer, have less disease, and feel better. They point out that it is exactly how much of the vitamins that start out in our foodstuffs are still there after they are ground up, frozen, shipped thousands of miles, cooked, canned, stocked on store shelves, and then put down before us on our dinner plates.

While the experts joust over the minutiae of their vitamin test results, Americans are voting with their pocketbooks for the side that advocates taking extra vitamins in pills and capsules. The latest figures show sales of multivitamins growing at almost 20 percent a year, vitamin E sales are growing at 30 percent, and sales of beta-carotene, an antioxidant nutrient that the body can make into vitamin A, are growing at about 20 percent. Altogether, the American public spends over three billion dollars annually on dietary supplements.

Unabashedly, this book sides with those who favor taking vitamins. As such, it should serve as your guide to what vitamins you should consider taking, which nutrients you should avoid, what dosages and formulations seem to be the most beneficial, and what kind of information to watch out for as new vitamin studies appear in the media.

Along the way, I've included some nutritional history so you can better understand how our knowledge of nutrition grew to be what it is today. As you will see, the conflicting advice from nutrition researchers reported in the media over what to eat and drink is not a new phenomenon. Nutrition controversy accompanied the very first discoveries of the nutrients in food. There are parallels between the way the public ignores diet advice today and the way it always has, even when the advice has the potential for saving thousands of lives.

Finally, as I make clear in this book, taking vitamins should not be considered a panacea for what ails you or for what you think might ail you someday. Taking vitamins should be part of an overall healthy lifestyle. Vitamins should not be looked upon as a cure for being overweight, not getting enough exercise, or eating a high-fat, nutrient-poor diet. To get the most benefit from vitamins, you should plan a mostly vegetarian diet that goes easy on meat, soft drinks, alcoholic beverages, and gooey desserts. Fresh vegetarian foods are full of vitamins and other nutrients that are vital to optimal health. Many of the nutrients in vegetables that may be important for forestalling cancer, heart disease, and other conditions are not well understood if they are even known at all. The majority of these substances are not available in any pill, capsule, or supplement. You have to eat them in food.

Despite our paucity of information about many of the mysterious nutrients lurking in our salads and vegetables, it is still possible to plan a reliable supplement program to go along with a healthy diet. There are definite guidelines you can follow, although many of the supplement rules allow flexibility. A lot of what you finally decide to take depends on your individual needs and how supplements make you feel. Of course, as I point out, there are nutrients you need to be wary of, nutrients which, in high doses, may cause medical problems. But most vitamins are quite safe in substantial amounts and, within a reasonable range, you can make up your own mind about your body's needs.

1

Getting Started

Many books on vitamins, diet, and nutrition make glowing promises that sound too good to be true. They herald long life, clear complexions, and endless personal energy if only you follow the advice hidden in the glowingly titled chapters. Unfortunately, there's a catch to these miraculous claims. They lack factual evidence to back them up. No scientific proof has been found that shows eating certain foods or taking nutritional supplements will make bald heads grow hair, cause gray hair to turn back to its original color, make cancer vanish, or drastically improve your looks.

This book makes no fantastic or outlandish claims for vitamins or any other nutrients. It doesn't have to. Now there is a sufficient number of factually based— and equally impressive—benefits of vitamins to suit anyone's fancy. The rapidly progressing field of nutrition research has been finding powerful vitamin health benefits worthy enough of any health-minded person's attention. Even if vitamins won't make you look like a movie star, their health boosting powers are still cause for applause.

PR for Vitamins

Anyone with a television set or magazine subscription surely realizes that research into the health effects of vitamins is accelerating rapidly. Rarely does a month go by without a report of a new study heralding the health benefits of one or more vitamins. That's because, within the last few years, many segments of the health establishment have discovered vitamins in a big way. Consequently, researchers are compiling more and more evidence that taking extra vitamins in the form of supplements is most probably very beneficial to health, well-being, and longevity.

As you may recall, the American mainstream medical world was not always so hospitable to the thought that vitamin supplements could be good for you. Some parts of the establishment still aren't, but the number of skeptics is diminishing with every new study. Just a few years ago, virtually all conservative medical people talked down the benefits of vitamins. At the same time, they also resisted the idea that diet had a large effect on health. As a result, in many people's minds, vitamins became inextricably linked to health-food faddism and hocus-pocus nutrition.

By now, of course, it is universally accepted that the food you eat affects your wellness. However, there is still entrenched opposition to the idea that vitamin pills can improve health, despite the growing piles of research papers showing just that.

High Profit Medicine

Why have so many experts ridiculed the notion that taking doses of vitamins could be healthy?

Sadly, a large part of the blame has to go to the very structure of American medicine. Too often, therapies and treatments that provide large profit margins seem to inexorably draw the approval of doctors, pharmaceutical companies, and medical equipment manufacturers. These same groups feed the media press releases extolling high-tech medicine, and they hire experts whose opinions are reprinted in the nation's newspapers. In this profit-oriented environment there is often relatively little information available about generic substances such as vitamins that cannot be patented and sold exclusively at the kind of substantial profits generated by new drugs.

Of course, it would be wrong to blame individual researchers and doctors for the attention given to high-tech, expensive medical treatments and the neglect of more benign, preventive tools such as nutrition. It is more a structural problem and a problem of perspective inherent in the health care delivery system. For the most part, modern American medicine has focused on the cure of acute medical conditions. Generally speaking, doctors have concentrated on curing serious problems afflicting their patients. They have had less knowledge about how to prevent the diseases their patients would get in the future. Often this orientation toward curing acute disease and neglecting preventive medicine still persists.

Doctors Don't Check Nutrition

Many news stories on health and nutrition refer readers to their doctors, but how concerned are doctors about the nutrients their patients consume? The answer is not reassuring. In one nationwide survey of physicians, researchers discovered that most doctors never bother to check to see what kind of nutrition their patients get either in their diets or their vitamin supplements. As a matter of fact, this survey revealed that not even doctors who had taken nutrition courses in medical school or physicians professing a belief in the importance of nutrition advise their patients on how to get proper nutrition that would help them stay healthy.

The study, which looked at the nutrition orientation of more than 3,400 doctors, was a mail-in survey to which only about one in ten doctors responded. We can conclude that the nonrespondents—the majority of doctors—were probably even less concerned about nutrition than the physicians who answered the questionnaires.

The survey revealed that your chances of having a doctor who talks to you about nutrition are better if the doctor you are seeing has actually made an improvement in her/his own diet. In that case, the doctor is more likely to have some curiosity about what you are eating and is more likely to give you some advice about how to improve your dietary profile. Apparently, doctors' personal involvement with nutrition translates into an increase in involvement with their patients' eating habits. Interestingly enough, the study also showed that doctors who had gone to school in foreign countries were more likely to talk to their patients about the importance of nutrition.

On the negative side, even though younger doctors and doctors who had taken at least one nutrition course in medical school had a more open-minded attitude about the importance of diet and nutrition as being factors that influence health, these physicians were no more likely to advise patients about nutrition than were other doctors.

Pregnancy and Vitamins

Perhaps the most important time to be concerned about vitamins and nutrition is when you are pregnant. The nutrition of about-to-be-pregnant and pregnant women is vital for the health of the developing fetus as well as for women bearing children. Researchers now believe that some birth defects are caused or influenced by poor maternal nutrition. In particular, several large studies have shown that neural tube defects—serious malformations of the fetal nervous system—are most probably directly attributable to a lack of a B vitamin called folate.

Expectant fathers should not be complacent about their vitamin status, either. There is evidence demonstrating that the amount of vitamin C a would-be father takes in may have an effect on the health of his sperm.

Despite the fact that mothers and fathers should eat a high-quality diet (and probably should take vitamins) before, during, and after pregnancy, a survey of obstetricians and gynecologists found that doctors "rarely see their patients before pregnancy and not before the fourth week of pregnancy." That may be too late. Nutrition's most important influence on fetal development probably takes place right around the time of conception.

The good news, though, is that the doctors reported almost always prescribing vitamins for pregnant women. These vitamins are prenatal multivitamins including folic acid and the minerals iron and calcium. Aside from that nutrition prescription, the doctors rarely asked the women about the number of calories they were eating or how nutritious their diets were. In addition, they believed their pregnant patients could get all the nutrients they required from food and had no need for vitamin supplements. Apparently the vitamins they prescribed were an insurance policy in case they were wrong about this belief.

How current were these doctors with the latest nutritional research? The report found that these physicians had not changed their nutritional recommendations at any time during the past five years, a finding that's not too reassuring in the light of all the nutrition discoveries that are taking place every year.

All of this means that you, as a medical consumer— pregnant or not—better know a bit about nutrition for your own self-interest, since it's likely that your doctor is not going to be very well-informed about nutrition and will not ask you about the food you've been eating, the beverages you've been drinking, or the vitamin pills you've been taking.

The Myth of the Balanced Diet

If you can't depend on a doctor's advice about nutrition and vitamins, whose advice can you depend on? That's not an easy question to answer. Within the past ten years, the vast amount of nutrition research that has gone on has yielded startling discoveries that have put the whole field of nutrition in flux and called into question some of the field's most cherished long-standing precepts. As we'll see, this is not a new state of affairs for nutrition science. Throughout its history, the science of diet and nutrition has been a constant battlefield of opposing viewpoints, periodically revolutionized by research that contradicted what nutrition scientists thought they knew about the human body.

Until very recently, the vast majority of nutrition experts have insisted that the average, healthy person should not take vitamin supplements. The establishment view held that you could get all of the vitamins and nutrients you needed from a healthy diet. In many places, this point of view still prevails. However, the ranks of the defectors who recognize the value of vitamin supplements are growing as large studies demonstrate vitamin benefits.

Do the Right Thing

I, too, used to believe in the myth of the balanced diet. As a health writer who specialized in nutrition, I believed that if you ate a wide variety of fruits and vegetables, ate meat only in moderation, got a reasonable amount of exercise, and kept your weight at a desirable level, you were doing all you could for good health. With the proper diet, so it seemed, there was no need to take vitamin pills. They were an unnecessary waste of money for nutrients that passed through your body without making any difference to your health. This was what many of the experts I consulted told me. I had taken vitamins for a while in my twenties and thirties and then had given them up.

For me, for a while, giving up vitamins seemed to be an acceptable course of action. My health seemed good. I jogged about twenty miles a week, every week. I rarely got a cold. I looked and felt fine, or so I thought.

Even though my health seemed to be excellent, my body hid a deadly surprise. In my early forties I started to experience breathing problems when I ran. It was nothing major, just a slight tug in my chest that would consistently make itself felt after I was about half a mile into my daily run of three miles. Since my breathing discomfort usually dissipated after a few minutes of relaxed jogging, I assumed I was suffering exercise induced asthma, constriction of the bronchial tubes brought on by exertion. But the breathing difficulty was persistent, and it appeared almost every time I exercised.

My breathing problem started around Thanksgiving of my forty-second year and continued throughout the winter into the early spring. At Christmas that year, I also experienced a serious case of the flu that kept me in bed for two weeks.

During that February I started a stressful job—a job at a book publishing company in which I was required to manage thirty different projects at the same time. I found the tasks at the job daunting. I felt extremely pressured as I tried to keep track of manuscripts that were traveling across the country to freelance copyeditors in Pennsylvania, being illustrated by artists in New Jersey, revised by authors in Maine, indexed in New York, and rewritten in Connecticut. My breathing problems grew worse. What had been a mild tug that started about four minutes into my daily runs had now become a persistent ache at three minutes or less.

In June, after a four mile run that was an agony of chest discomfort, I finally went to my family doctor. By this time, I suspected I was having a serious problem. I could think of no other explanation for the generalized ache that spread through my chest and arms while I was running except that I must be having heart problems.

My family doctor poked and prodded me and told me I was suffering exercise induced asthma. After all, he insisted, I was in good physical shape, slim, had been regularly running for almost twenty years, and ate a decent diet. Still, since I was over forty, he sent me to a cardiologist for an exercise stress test.

On the treadmill in the cardiologist's office, hooked up to a heart monitor, I flunked the stress test dramatically. Further, invasive medical tests showed that one of the arteries feeding blood to my heart was almost completely blocked. There was a good chance that without treatment, this artery, known both as the left anterior descending artery and also as the "widowmaker," soon would have blocked up completely, killing me with a massive heart attack.

The day after my forty-third birthday, I had my artery

opened up with a procedure known as angioplasty, an operation that involves feeding an expandable balloon catheter through arteries in the leg, past the heart, to the blockage, and pushing the coronary artery open. Three months after the first one of these procedures, the artery became reblocked (reoccluded) and had to be reopened.

Why did this heart problem happen to me after years of exercising, eating right, and watching my weight and cholesterol? Aside from the fact that heart disease runs in my family, I firmly believe that the fact that I didn't take extra vitamins—particularly the antioxidant vitamins C and E and beta-carotene—influenced the development of my disease. While exercise builds up the muscles of your arms and legs and your heart muscles, it also generates destructive molecules known as free radicals, which can damage various parts of the body and can contribute to blockages of your arteries (see page 33). Recent studies indicate that the antioxidant vitamins can help prevent this damage and work against the buildup of plaque, the material that impedes blood flow and causes arteriosclerosis.

I often wonder what would have happened to me if I had not stopped taking vitamins in my thirties. Would my disease still have progressed to the point where it threatened my life? There is no way to know with any kind of certainty what vitamins would have done for me. I do know that since beginning a new vitamin regimen, my artery has stayed clear and I have stopped suffering angina, the painful ache in my chest that results when a blocked artery prevents the heart from receiving a sufficient blood supply.

I also know that in scientific terms, my experience would not convince a scientist of the value of vitamin supplementation. The conventional medical wisdom claims that my becoming a victim of heart disease at the age of forty-three had nothing to do with vitamins. I don't believe it, because I do know that following all of the approved methods of preventing heart disease didn't work for me.

Diet Plus Vitamins

Despite my experience in developing heart disease while eating what is supposed to be a heart-healthy diet (low in fat, high in carbohydrates), I still believe in the importance of being careful about what I eat. If my diet had included a higher amount of fat, perhaps I would have developed heart disease even sooner. Certainly, what you eat has a large influence on your health, whether you take vitamins or not.

Most importantly, in this there is virtually unanimous agreement among nutrition experts: No matter how effective they are, vitamin pills are *supplements*. That means that they can supplement or add to the nutrition of a good diet, but they are not substitutes. They will never substitute for eating the right foods and they cannot rectify poor health habits such as smoking or drinking too much alcohol or overindulging in fatty or sugary foods.

It is also important to keep in mind that it can be dangerous to diagnose your own serious medical problems and try to treat them yourself with diet or vitamins. If you believe you are suffering any kind of serious medical condition, see your doctor. Vitamins and diet are important for preventing disease and promoting wellness, but only rarely can they be used to treat illness, and even when they are, you should be under the care of a competent physician.

2

The RDA:
Nutrition by Committee

In examining our requirements for vitamins, nutrition experts constantly refer to the RDA, the recommended dietary allowances. These numbers represent the basic vitamin intakes that the Food and Nutrition Board of the National Research Council has determined Americans should consume daily to maintain their health. From the RDA is derived the USRDA, more general numbers pertaining to daily nutrient intake that is supposed to be appropriate for food and supplement labels. While RDA recommendations for nutrient intake are broken down into gender and age groups (for instance, men over the age of fifty-five have different RDAs than women under the age of twenty-four, USRDAs are more generalized amounts applicable to just about everyone. As of this writing, the Food and Drug Administration has proposed a new set of standards, the RDI, which would basically replace the USRDA.

Origin of the RDA

Ever since 1941, the recommended dietary allowances (RDAs) have been drawn up by a committee known as the Food and Nutrition Board. The RDA list includes

Category	Age (years) or Condition	Weight[b] (kg)	(lb)	Height[b] (cm)	(in)	Protein (g)	Fat-Soluble Vitamins Vitamin A (μg RE)[c]	Vitamin D (μg)[d]	Vitamin E (mg α-TE)[e]	Vitamin K (μg)
Infants	0.0–0.5	6	13	60	24	13	375	7.5	3	5
	0.5–1.0	9	20	71	28	14	375	10	4	10
Children	1–3	13	29	90	35	16	400	10	6	15
	4–6	20	44	112	44	24	500	10	7	20
	7–10	28	62	132	52	28	700	10	7	30
Males	11–14	45	99	157	62	45	1,000	10	10	45
	15–18	66	145	176	69	59	1,000	10	10	65
	19–24	72	160	177	70	58	1,000	10	10	70
	25–50	79	174	176	70	63	1,000	5	10	80
	51+	77	170	173	68	63	1,000	5	10	80
Females	11–14	46	101	157	62	46	800	10	8	45
	15–18	55	120	163	64	44	800	10	8	55
	19–24	58	128	164	65	46	800	10	8	60
	25–50	63	138	163	64	50	800	5	8	65
	51+	65	143	160	63	50	800	5	8	65
Pregnant						60	800	10	10	65
Lactating	1st 6 months					65	1,300	10	12	65
	2nd 6 months					62	1,200	10	11	65

[a] The allowances, expressed as average daily intakes over time, are intended to provide for individual variations among most normal persons as they live in the United States under usual environmental stresses. Diets should be based on a variety of common foods in order to provide other nutrients for which human requirements have been less well defined. See text for detailed discussion of allowances and of nutrients not tabulated.

[b] Weights and heights of Reference Adults are actual medians for the U.S. population of the designated age, as reported by NHANES II. The median weights and heights of those under 19 years of age were taken from Hamill et al. (1979) (see pages 16–17). The use of these figures does not imply that the height-to-weight ratios are ideal.

vitamins, minerals, trace elements, carbohydrates, fats, and protein. The committee analyzes the latest nutrition research for each nutrient and records the amounts that it believes should be consumed on a daily basis by certain population groups, such as infants and children, as well as adult men and women. According to the board, these amounts are "the levels of intake of essential nutrients that, on the basis of scientific knowledge, are judged by the Food and Nutrition Board to be adequate to meet the known nutrient needs of practically all healthy persons."

The RDAs were originally an American wartime

Academy of Sciences—National Research Council
Allowances,[a] Revised 1989
of practically all healthy people in the United States

Water-Soluble Vitamins							Minerals						
Vitamin C (mg)	Thiamin (mg)	Riboflavin (mg)	Niacin (mg NE)[f]	Vitamin B6 (mg)	Folate (µg)	Vitamin B12 (µg)	Calcium (mg)	Phosphorus (mg)	Magnesium (mg)	Iron (mg)	Zinc (mg)	Iodine (µg)	Selenium (µg)
30	0.3	0.4	5	0.3	25	0.3	400	300	40	6	5	40	10
35	0.4	0.5	6	0.6	35	0.5	600	500	60	10	5	50	15
40	0.7	0.8	9	1.0	50	0.7	800	800	80	10	10	70	20
45	0.9	1.1	12	1.1	75	1.0	800	800	120	10	10	90	20
45	1.0	1.2	13	1.4	100	1.4	800	800	170	10	10	120	30
50	1.3	1.5	17	1.7	150	2.0	1,200	1,200	270	12	15	150	40
60	1.5	1.8	20	2.0	200	2.0	1,200	1,200	400	12	15	150	50
60	1.5	1.7	19	2.0	200	2.0	1,200	1,200	350	10	15	150	70
60	1.5	1.7	19	2.0	200	2.0	800	800	350	10	15	150	70
60	1.2	1.4	15	2.0	200	2.0	800	800	350	10	15	150	70
50	1.1	1.3	15	1.4	150	2.0	1,200	1,200	280	15	12	150	45
60	1.1	1.3	15	1.5	180	2.0	1,200	1,200	300	15	12	150	50
60	1.1	1.3	15	1.6	180	2.0	1,200	1,200	280	15	12	150	55
60	1.1	1.3	15	1.6	180	2.0	800	800	280	15	12	150	55
60	1.0	1.2	13	1.6	180	2.0	800	800	280	10	12	150	55
70	1.5	1.6	17	2.2	400	2.2	1,200	1,200	320	15	15	175	65
95	1.6	1.8	20	2.1	280	2.6	1,200	1,200	355	15	19	200	75
90	1.6	1.7	20	2.1	260	2.6	1,200	1,200	340	15	16	200	75

[c] Retinol equivalents. 1 retinol equivalent = 1 µg retinol or 6 µg β-carotene. See text for calculation of vitamin A activity of diets as retinol equivalents.

[d] As cholecalciferol. 10 µg cholecalciferol = 400 IU of vitamin D.

[e] α-Tocopherol equivalents. 1 mg d-α tocopherol = 1 α-TE. See text for variation in allowances and calculation of vitamin E activity of the diet as α-tocopherol equivalents.

[f] 1 NE (niacin equivalent) is equal to 1 mg of niacin or 60 mg of dietary tryptophan.

effort to construct a scientific yardstick measuring the nutrients people needed in their diets to survive. The federal government, afraid that food supplies might be limited during World War II, wanted to make sure that the food available would be sufficiently nutritious in case of an emergency.

The business of figuring out nutritional requirements was still a very young science when the RDAs were born. In the 1920s, the concept of overall nutritive requirements for a long list of substances began to win scientific recognition. In 1935, the Technical Committee on Nutrition of the League of

Nations made the first officially sanctioned attempt at coming up with nutrition recommendations. That first committee limited its recommendations to protein and calories.

From the very beginning, the task of determining official nutrient recommendations has been a belabored, bureaucratic affair. America's World War II effort started with a Committee on Foods and Nutrition that was set up within the Division of Biology and Agriculture in the National Academy of Sciences Research Council under the aegis of the Council on National Defense. As soon as all the bureaucrats were in place, these groups held a National Nutrition Conference in May of 1941 to get the ball rolling.

It's been rolling controversially ever since. As you might expect from anything derived by committee, the RDAs have generated a great deal of argument and debate ever since their inception. Even under the best circumstances, figures like the RDAs are only approximations of the nutrient levels that large numbers of healthy people should be consuming.

What's wrong with devising RDAs for healthy people? In some ways, these watered down nutrient prescriptions are the nutritional equivalent of the mythical all-American nuclear family. This stereotypical group doesn't really exist, but it is a comforting icon to hang onto.

The RDAs, in their own way, are the same kind of symbol. They are a comforting construct that assures us that Americans are getting most of their necessary nutrients from their food. Actually, some studies of the American diet show that many people don't even meet the modest levels of the RDAs. Although the RDA list of nutrients and numbers are designed for healthy people, no one really knows precisely what population group this refers to. These numbers merely represent a type of lowest common denominator for figuring out the amounts of vitamins and other nutrients that large numbers of people probably should be getting in their diets so as not to develop serious deficiency diseases, according to the committee that does the figuring.

As stated by Alfred E. Harper, Ph.D., who chaired the 1974 RDA committee, these allowances "are compatible with maintenance of the health of most people." According to a previous chairperson of the RDA committee, these figures are "goals at which to aim in providing for the nutritional needs of groups of people."

Note the emphasis on the fact that the RDAs are meant for groups of people, not for individuals. In other words, if you are trying to create a program of optimal nutrition for yourself, the RDAs may provide a basic measurement of nutrient levels you should surpass, but they are not a reliable guide for what you should optimally consume in your diet or in vitamin supplements.

Obvious Signs of Deficiency

As Joan Dye Gussow, Ed.D., and Paul Thomas, M.S., R.D., point out in their book, *The Nutrition Debate,* the RDAs are meant to be the level of vitamins and nutrients people need in order to be safe from "obvious signs of deficiency." What the RDAs miss are signs of deficiency that are subtle and not easily detected. For instance, Americans suffer from an epidemic of heart disease. Could this partly reflect the fact that they are suffering from a lack of antioxidant vitamins that could preserve their heart health? Couldn't that fact, at least in part, be theorized as a deficiency disease?

Dr. Linus Pauling, winner of two Nobel prizes and a relentless advocate for the benefits of taking massive amounts of vitamin C, claims "the RDA [is supposed to be] the amount needed to keep the average person in ordinary good health. I say it keeps them in ordinary bad health."

Even if the RDA was sufficient for good health, the truth is that few Americans eat a balanced diet full of enough fruits and vegetables to meet every one of these minimal vitamin standards. Even if the average person were striving to eat a healthy diet, how would it be possible for someone to figure out how much vitamin C or E or beta-carotene she ate yesterday in her food? Most people, even those with advanced degrees in nutrition, have little idea exactly how much of the micronutrients they consume daily.

Added to this problem of calculating the micronutrients in your food is another perplexing factor: Large numbers of us are constantly limiting our food intake in order to lose weight. Often, when you are dieting, you are missing out on vitamins as well as calories. It is very difficult for dieters to fulfill the RDA for vitamins. It is so difficult, in fact, that even the most conservative nutritionists admit that dieters should take vitamin supplements. Women are especially at risk for not consuming enough vitamins, since their food intake is generally only about two-thirds that of men.

Aside from the influence of gender, it is safe to say that every individual has peculiar dietary needs that cannot be met by a generalized list like the RDA. Each of us has an individual genetic makeup that influences how much of each vitamin we need for good health. Each of us undergoes a different amount of stress that may deplete us of vitamins. A particularly modern problem is the amount of pollutants we encounter in our daily lives. The more pollutants you encounter in your home or at your job, the more vitamins you may need to keep your body healthy.

For instance, if your spouse smokes, your body will

require more vitamin C to offset the negative effects of the sidestream smoke you inhale. If you live in a large city where the air is constantly filled with smog, you should probably increase your daily consumption of vitamin E, which some researchers believe can help alleviate the deleterious influence of air pollution.

RDA Figures are Averages

The most important points to keep in mind about the RDA numbers are:

• The RDAs are guesses about the amounts of vitamins and other nutrients that are necessary to avoid extremely poor health. They do not reflect upper limits on what may be necessary for optimal health.

• The RDAs are numbers that reflect the overall nutritional needs of groups. They do not apply to individuals. Each of us may actually require less or more than the RDA for any particular nutrient.

• The RDAs do not take into account special circumstances that may require extra doses of particular vitamins. For instance, if you smoke, you will need extra doses of the antioxidant vitamins. Do not try to treat yourself for serious medical conditions, however. If you have a serious medical problem, consult your doctor.

History of Vitamins

Although much of the latest research into the functions of vitamins in the human body provides evidence that certain vitamin supplements will probably protect you from disease, many conservative nutritionists and medical people still insist that taking vitamin supplements is not necessary for good health. They insist that all the vitamins most people need can be consumed in a balanced diet.

This conservative point of view grows out of an anachronistic perspective that has its roots in the early history of vitamins and vitamin discovery. The very idea of vitamins, nutrients that are necessary in very small amounts for good health, was originally developed as a tool for fighting deficiency disease, not as a means of enhancing health. When conservative nutritionists and dietitians insist that most individuals don't need vitamin supplements, what they are actually saying is that they don't recognize that we may be suffering from vitamin deficiencies that are not readily identifiable. In their view, if you seem healthy or if you merely suffer from the chronic diseases that many Americans are prone to, then you don't need extra vitamins.

The most serious shortcoming of this viewpoint is that it fails to take into account the benefits of vitamins consumed above the level needed to stave off the obvious deficiency diseases. Just because we don't suffer from debilitating conditions like beriberi or pellagra does not necessarily mean we get an optimal level of vitamins in our diets.

Consider the history of scurvy, one of the first generally well-known vitamin deficiency diseases. Although we now know that this condition is caused by a lack of vitamin C, before the discovery of deficiency diseases, scurvy was a mysterious, deadly illness shrouded in mystery.

Scurvy was a particular danger to ocean sailors who consumed little fresh food and who subsisted on a diet of bread, salted meat, and other foodstuffs that lasted a long time in the hold of a ship. Unfortunately, these foods contain virtually no vitamin C. The lack of this vitamin made scurvy a deadly killer on long journeys.

Scurvy is a frightening condition. Early on, it causes feelings of listlessness, lack of strength, and exhaustion. As time goes on, scurvy victims suffer painful aches in the muscles. They feel depressed. Then their gums develop ulcers as their teeth fall out. Their muscles bruise as hemorrhages appear throughout the body. Finally, racked by diarrhea, lungs and kidneys give out and death soon follows.

On some long voyages, fatalities from scurvy outnumbered the survivors. When Vasco da Gama made a voyage in the 1490s from Portugal to India, only about 60 of his 160 sailors survived. The rest were killed by scurvy. Other sea captains had similar experiences.

It wasn't until the eighteenth century that Europeans accepted that scurvy could be cured by diet. At that time, a Scottish doctor named James Lind took twelve scurvy patients and fed them different diets to see if particular foods could cure the condition. Two of the patients received a daily ration of cider with their food. Two others were fed a dilute solution of sulfuric acid. Others were fed seawater. Still others were given vinegar, seawater, or medicine. Two received oranges and lemons every day.

Of course, since oranges and lemons are citrus fruits containing vitamin C, at the end of the experiment these last two lucky patients recovered while the other men remained sick. Lind wrote up the results of his studies in a book called *A Treatise on Scurvy,* which he published in 1753.

Interestingly enough, more than two hundred years before Lind carried out his experiments, Native Americans had offered a cure for scurvy to European explorers, but this knowledge had generally been ignored. In the 1530s, a Frenchman, Jacques Cartier, sailed up what is now known as the Saint Lawrence River and wintered near what is now the Canadian city of Quebec. While they were there, many of Cartier's sailors suffered from scurvy and about two dozen of them died. Local Native Americans, taking pity on the suffering Europeans, showed Cartier that drinking tea from the bark and leaves of the spruce tree would alleviate scurvy. Modern day measurements show that this tea is fairly high in vitamin C.

It seems to take a long time for denizens of Western civilization to accept dietary changes and good nutrition advice. Even after Lind's experiments, not everyone accepted the premise that scurvy could be cured with citrus fruit. One who did was Captain James Cook, who made long voyages from England to the Pacific in the 1760s and 1770s. He found that feeding his crews fresh food as often as possible was beneficial to their health. His sailors believed that fresh food not only kept them from getting scurvy but also prevented colds. He always stocked his ships with sauerkraut, another food containing vitamin C.

It wasn't until 1795—almost fifty years after Lind carried out his research—that the British Admiralty ordered its captains to feed sailors lime juice to prevent scurvy, and it wasn't until the middle of the nineteenth century, in 1865 that the British merchant marine was ordered to provide lime juice. No one knows how many sailors died from lack of vitamin C while the British bureaucrats delayed passing these regulations.

Today, of course, few people in the United States suffer from acute symptoms of scurvy. However, one nutrition expert has pointed out, only half in jest, that if it weren't for the meager amount of vitamin C in fast food French fried potatoes, many children and a large proportion of adults would be consuming no vitamin C in their diet and scurvy would once again become common.

Some nutritionists believe that our willful disregard for what we should be eating for optimal health bears a similarity to what went on in Lind's time. Today, as in Lind's era, vitamin and nutrition research has progressed faster than the medical establishment's ability to shift perspective. The standard position that a balanced diet will supply all the vitamins that a healthy person needs does not adequately acknowledge the latest scientific findings.

In the field of nutrition, many scientists pride themselves on being slow to change their minds. They believe that this reticence protects them from being the victims of faddish discoveries that will eventually be disproven. That attitude is surely mistaken in the face of evidence that large doses of vitamins and other nutrients—especially vitamin C, vitamin E, and beta-carotene—can protect the human body against aging, heart disease, cancer, and other debilitating conditions. Still, these scientists insist on waiting until all the evidence is in.

Luckily for you, if you are concerned about giving yourself the optimal intake of vitamins, you don't have to wait until all the evidence is in. Since you can take vitamin supplements at levels that certainly will do no harm, it's a smart bet to take them and try to reap the health benefits. Countless experiments have shown that these vitamins are safe. Even though some experts insist that the only thing vitamin supplements can accomplish is to give you expensive urine when you excrete what your body can't use, the possible good you will be doing yourself makes vitamins a good bet.

3

The Antioxidant Vitamins

Rust Never Sleeps

Much of the recent research into the benefits of vitamins has focused on the nutrients known as antioxidants. Scientists are only now coming to grips with the large role that antioxidants play in preventing disease. Consequently, not many people understand what antioxidants are or what they do.

The ideas behind the theories of how antioxidants function in our bodies are not that hard to understand or use to your advantage. Put in simplest terms, this area of nutrition research demonstrates that vitamins A, C, and E and beta-carotene, as well as other antioxidant nutrients, protect your cells from diseases like cancer and arteriosclerosis by nullifying the destructive power of molecules called free radicals. If unchecked, free radicals are reactive substances that wreak havoc with cell structures.

Through research in this area, scientists have come to realize that oxygen—a gas you breathe every moment of your life—often creates caustic by-products that can destroy the life it sustains.

Oxygen: Breath of Life and Destroyer

A constant supply of oxygen, of course, is necessary for human life. To prove that, you merely have to hold your breath for a few moments and witness your body's urgent reaction. Although that desperate desire to breathe is stimulated by the level of carbon dioxide in your blood (carbon dioxide is a waste product of the respiration in each of your cells), it is the oxygen that you inhale that allows your metabolism—and your life—to continue.

Metabolism is a catchall word that refers to the energy-consuming processes going on in your body at all times. Your body requires energy to build new tissues, fuel activity, and maintain the well-being of all its cells. You couldn't lift a finger and your body could not heal a cut without it. These metabolic processes of repair and movement almost always require oxygen.

To the human body, as well as to all plants and animals, oxygen is something to defend against as well as to use. It is a highly reactive substance. When it plays a part in controlled reactions in your body, it liberates useful energy. If it is allowed to react without constraint, it has the capability of destroying tissues wholesale and wreaking havoc during normal cellular activities. This destructive power mostly derives from by-products of your body's metabolic use of oxygen, which liberates what are called free radicals. In your body, free radicals are rogue molecules that chemically react with cell structures and other substances. These reactions are believed to initiate or promote diseases such as cancer, heart disease, and emphysema. They are also thought to play an important role in aging. Many scientists believe that free radicals' destructive oxidative actions are important factors that are involved in everything from arthritis to the formation of wrinkles as we grow old.

Oxidation, the reaction of oxygen with other chemicals, is the process that causes metals to rust, wood to burn, and sliced apples to turn brown. As a matter of fact, if you coat a sliced apple with an antioxidant such as vitamin C, the vitamin C slows the oxidative reactions, and the apple will take longer to change color. When oxidative chemicals in your body run rampant, they can cause the cellular version of rust. Your body constantly defends against this destruction through the use of special protective mechanisms and with antioxidant vitamins, if they are available.

Free Radicals' Electron Danger

The oxidative substances in the body that most often present a health danger are called free radicals because they are electrically charged pieces of molecules—radicals—that have broken loose in the protoplasm and are ready to react destructively with whatever cellular structures they contact. The electrical charge of these molecular fragments results from the extra electrons the radical possesses or lacks. When electrons are paired, as they are in most of the substances in your body, they tend to stay at home and not cause trouble. The unpaired electrons in free radicals have a tendency to jump to other molecules or claim electrons from those other molecules. This exchange of electrons, which, in the chemist's parlance, is another form of oxidation, disrupts the cell's normal activities.

Because of their unstable and reactive nature, free radicals are the anarchistic terrorists of the cell. Their reactions can alter genes, causing unwanted genetic mutations. Free radicals can also latch onto and alter cell membranes. At this time, when they react with a neighboring molecule, say, by discharging an extra electron, they sometimes start a brutal chain reaction that destroys a whole host of other molecules.

As you might expect, the human body has evolved many defenses against this destruction as well as methods for repairing the resultant damage. One notorious, frequently formed free radical, a chemical called superoxide, is so dangerous that the body has developed a complex system of unique enzymes solely to defuse its destructive power. When this chemical appears inside the body, first an enzyme called superoxide dismutase tackles superoxide and transforms it into hydrogen peroxide. This is followed up by a reaction with catalase, another enzyme, that changes the hydrogen peroxide into water and a stable, harmless, and metabolically usable form of oxygen.

Within the cellular antioxidant defense mechanisms, there are also specialized protective systems designed to protect DNA, the genetic material that directs the activities of the protoplasm. Harm to the cell's DNA can be the most lethal form of destruction, since damaged DNA often leaves cells vulnerable to cancer or cell death. But there are enzymes that can recognize when DNA has suffered oxidative damage and repair the damaged areas.

Scientists who have studied free radicals believe that when their damage builds up over time or increases so much that the body can't keep up with the destruction, serious disease is the result. Plus, when people get old, it is believed that their repair mechanisms may stop working efficiently, making them more vulnerable to conditions such as arthritis, heart disease, and cancer.

Taking antioxidant vitamins supplies your body with extra tools for fighting off these destructive reactions.

While scientists are far from finished with their exploration of this field, the evidence gathered so far indicates that beta-carotene and vitamins C and E provide powerful ammunition for decreasing the harmful effects of free radicals.

Brain Protection

Based on the theories of how free radicals work in the body, evidence has been found that shows that antioxidants play an important role in protecting the brain. They are apparently crucial for minimizing brain damage that results from strokes. Studies looking into what happens when brain tissue loses its blood supply during a stroke find that most of the destruction of brain cells that results in paralysis or memory loss does not take place while the blood supply is interrupted. It actually occurs when the blood flows back in as the stroke ends. As the blood surges back through the vessels, the oxidative reactions of free radicals increases greatly. The presence of antioxidants can curtail some of this damage.

In studies on animals, researchers have discovered that older animals suffer more oxidative brain damage than do younger ones. In one experiment that examined the effects of oxidation on performance, a drug called PBN (alpha-phenyl-N-tert-butyl nitrone) was used to stimulate the animals' brains to produce enzymes that fight off free radical oxidative damage. After getting the drug, the animals performed better in finding their way through mazes, indicating that antioxidants such as these enzymes improve brain function.

What this suggests is that if you're smart (and want to stay that way), taking antioxidant vitamins now may help stave off free radical damage to your brain. It isn't absolute proof that this is true, but it's one more reason for supposing that these vitamins will keep you healthier as you age.

Aerobic Lifestyle: It Needs Protection

Strong evidence also shows that athletic performance may be aided by antioxidant vitamins. These vitamins are especially useful to those who indulge in strenuous aerobic exercise. As a matter of fact, that may be when you need antioxidant vitamins the most.

As reported in *Science News,* several studies have found that, although exercise stimulates your cardio-vascular system into becoming more efficient in using oxygen, the extra oxygen your body uses during exercise may result in tissue damage. Muscle tissue is particularly vulnerable to the oxidative processes that take place.

In one study, researchers at Ithaca College in Ithaca, New York, examined levels of the chemical malondialdehyde (MDA) in the urine of women who exercised on a treadmill. The excretion of this chemical is a sign that muscle is being oxidized. After half an hour on the treadmill, MDA levels in the exercisers rose by about a third. When the women took 400 IU (international units) of vitamin E every day, researchers found that after the women sweated it out in the gym, MDA levels fell by 28 percent instead of rising. The researchers concluded that antioxidant vitamins may actually reverse the oxidative stress that occurs during exercise.

Meanwhile, in Australia, other researchers who studied athletes from a variety of sports have come to the same basic conclusion. In this case, scientists gathered a dozen triathletes, long distance runners, and cross-country skiers at an Australian Olympic training center for a month and gave them pills to take every day before their workouts. Six of the athletes were given a daily pill containing 1,000

IU of vitamin E combined with a gram of vitamin C. The other athletes were fed placebos, similarly tasting pills that only contained sugar. Neither group knew which type of pill it was taking.

By studying the levels of two different enzymes in the athletes' blood, the researchers deduced that those who took the antioxidant vitamins displayed signs that their tissue oxidation had declined by 25 percent. These results support the idea that taking antioxidant vitamins can protect muscle tissue, including the muscle tissue of the heart, from oxidative stress that occurs during exercise. The researchers also felt that the vitamin supplements could protect red blood cells from damage.

On top of that, the Australian group found that these vitamins may protect athletes from overtraining. Training so hard that their performance suffers causes athletes to be more vulnerable to injury and stress. Overtrained athletes often feel tired and burnt out and their mental outlook usually suffers. Most often, athletes who suffer from training too vigorously have to take time off to recover.

In order to accurately determine the vitamins' effect on overtraining, the researchers measured the ratio of testosterone to cortisol in the athletes' blood. The ratio of these two hormones shifts when athletes overtrain: Testosterone decreases in overall relation to cortisol. The researchers found that the hard-training athletes who took vitamins C and E had increased ratios of testosterone to cortisol, a sign that the supplements were helping them reach higher levels of fitness without overstressing themselves. Because of this benefit, the athletes found they could train harder and perform better without feeling overtraining's ill effects.

Free Radicals and Heart Disease

The Australian researchers' data that indicated anti-oxidant vitamins may protect the heart from oxidative damage during exercise fits neatly into theories that protection from free radicals is important for the good health of your cardiovascular system. It is only within the past few years that researchers have begun to look into the possibility that free radicals are involved in the development of heart disease. Several recent studies in this area have shown that antioxidant drugs as well as antioxidant vitamins may help keep your arteries and blood-pumping machinery operating smoothly.

In spite of all the studies on heart disease, however, no one yet knows the exact mechanisms that set this disease in motion.

It is well known that cholesterol circulating in the blood is implicated in the formation of arterial blockages that damage the cardiovascular system and impair its function. Exactly how and why these buildups of plaque begin and progress until they dangerously block the flow of blood is still not well understood.

There is more than one type of cholesterol present in the blood. These lipoproteins (special combinations of fat and protein) that travel through the bloodstream can be classified as high-density lipoproteins (HDLs) and low-density lipoproteins (LDLs). To put it simply, HDLs are considered beneficial, but a high level of LDLs is associated with heart disease. HDLs usually transport cholesterol to the liver where it is broken down into other substances. LDLs, on the other hand, can deposit cholesterol on the artery walls, hindering circulation and causing the blockages of arteriosclerosis.

"One of the most perplexing questions in heart disease research has been determining the initial injury that begins the atherosclerotic process," says David Kritchevsky, Ph.D., associate director of the Wistar Institute of Anatomy and Biology in Philadelphia.

In the past, it has been believed that something occurs in the artery that damages the artery wall. Researchers felt that the buildup of cholesterol plaque at the site of damage might be the body's attempt to cover up the damaged area.

In Dr. Kritchevsky's view (supported by other researchers), it is most likely that the initial arterial injury is due to oxidation of the fatty acids contained in the blood's LDLs. According to this theory, hardening of the arteries begins when white blood cells known as monocytes stick to arterial walls. These monocytes then travel through the arterial walls and become macrophages, a special type of scavenger cell that filters material from fluid-filled spaces outside of the bloodstream.

Normally, this scavenging activity might not cause problems, but when the scavengers pick up oxidized LDLs, they are transformed into what are called foam cells, structures that begin a destructive chain of events that distort the artery and impede blood flow. The foam cells become bloated with fat globules and start a monocyte traffic jam, keeping other monocytes from slipping back out into the bloodstream. This jam-up of cells chemically encourages other scavengers to pick up oxidized LDL and turn into sluggish foam cells. Over time, the foam cell buildup creates plaque and damages cells in the artery walls. When the plaque bulges out into the artery, it impedes the flow of blood and can cause life-threatening blood clots.

By its overwhelming presence, the development of plaque also distorts muscular control of the artery. Normally, arteries are flexible, bending and stretching to accommodate rising and dropping blood flow. Plaque hinders this action, leaving the artery prone to painful and dangerous spasms. When a coronary artery feeding the heart closes in one of these spasms, the cut-off of the blood supply may cause a heart attack.

Apparently, the oxidation that may start this process doesn't just affect LDLs. Further research on this topic at Kyoto University in Japan shows that HDLs can be harmed by oxidation as well. Usually, it is believed, HDL can fight against the buildup of arterial plaque by taking cholesterol out of foam cells and transporting it to the liver where it can be converted into harmless substances that are eliminated from the body. However, Japanese researchers found evidence suggesting that oxidized HDL may have its cholesterol-transporting power compromised. When the HDL transport system breaks down, the clogging process that lays down plaque may accelerate.

In this complicated progression of events, the key preventive measure that may stave off heart disease is to stop the oxidation of HDLs and LDLs before plaque begins to form. If cholesterol can be saved from oxidation, then oxidized LDLs won't be absorbed by monocytes and used to form foam cells. Dr. Kritchevsky believes that nutrition may help protect LDLs from being oxidized by providing vitamins to soak up the oxidative power of free radicals.

The level of antioxidant vitamins dissolved in the blood may be a vital factor in protecting cholesterol from oxidation. When vitamin C is floating around in high quantities, it may preferentially react with the free radicals and nullify their destructive potential before they get a chance to destructively alter the LDLs and HDLs.

In addition to the protection afforded by the vitamin C circulating in the blood, LDL carries around its own arsenal of fat-soluble antioxidant molecules to protect its fatty acids. This self-contained protection consisting of beta-carotene and vitamin E can also keep the LDL fatty acids from being oxidized as long as the vitamin arsenal is well stocked.

If this theory of antioxidant protection is correct, taking vitamin E, beta-carotene, and vitamin C supplements so they can work their protective magic in your arteries will soon be widely recommended as preventive medicine against heart disease.

Weapons in the Heart Disease Battle

The medical establishment has traditionally relied on powerful drugs to battle cardiovascular disease, but a study at the University of Texas Southwestern Medical Center demonstrates that vitamin C may work better at preventing LDL oxidation than some pharmaceuticals. In this experiment (done in a test tube) vitamin C was found to decrease LDL absorption by monocytes by 93 percent while vitamin E cut the LDL uptake by 45 percent. A drug called probucol also prevented much of the LDL from being taken in by monocytes, but it did not protect the LDL's vitamin E and beta-carotene from being oxidized. The vitamin C, on the other hand, did protect the LDL's antioxidants.

Antioxidant Vitamins Fight Cancer

Research into antioxidants is building a strong case that these nutrients can fight cancer. As scientists better understand the various stages of cancer development, they are finding that a lack of these nutrients may make our bodies more vulnerable to the rapid multiplication of cancerous cells.

The situation is not simple, however. Cancer is not a single disease but a complex collection of diseases each characterized by a rampant, disorganized, uncontrolled proliferation of cells. In the worst cases of cancer, cells divide rapidly, never even reaching their mature stage as they invade and destroy tissues and organs. As is the case for virtually every disease, preventing cancer is preferable to trying to treat it once it occurs. In probing into the causes and development of cancer, researchers are discovering that oxidative destruction by free radicals may initiate this disease's development.

Most cancers progress in stages. After precancerous growths or lesions begin somewhere in the body due to a genetic malfunction or environmental insult, other stages have to occur before cells begin to reproduce uncontrollably and form what can be classified as cancerous tumors.

Normally, about ten million cells in your body reproduce every minute of your life. That means that in the next sixty seconds, between the time you begin this sentence and the moment you finish this paragraph, ten million of your cells will divide into twenty million new ones. If this reproduction takes place in an orderly fashion, your DNA, the genetic material contained within the nucleus of each cell, will control this process so that each new cell grows into a mature, properly functioning unit. When cancer strikes, cells divide rapidly, remain immature, and never fulfill their intended function. Instead, they mass together into tumors that can invade and fatally damage organs and tissues.

The Stages of Cancer

Researchers theorize that the shift from a normal cell to a cancerous cell doesn't happen in one simple step but usually takes place over a long period of time in several stages. The first stage is called initiation. It is believed that during initiation, something occurs that damages or changes the cell's genetic code or other basic cell structure. This change or mutation makes the cell more vulnerable to other cancer-causing factors called promoters. If, during the life of the cell that has been initiated, no other promoters are present, the cell will never become cancerous.

However, during the next stage, called promotion (or the latency period) if certain fats, hormones, or other agents of change interact with the cell, the cell can be converted into a much more dangerous precancerous state. In the case of many of the common cancers, this latency period can drag on from ten to thirty or even forty years.

If the cell enters the final stage of cancer, it is said to be in progression. It is at this point that cells reproduce in an uncontrollable fashion and form colonies (tumors) of malignant cells that destroy normal tissue. At this point, billions of cancer cells can be created. When these out-of-control cells journey through the blood or lymph system and invade various parts of the body, breaking off from the original cancer site, they are said to metastasize. This is the most dangerous stage of cancer because new, deadly tumors can form in virtually any organ of the body.

Medical researchers have not known much about how to prevent these stages from occurring, but they are beginning to understand more about the oxidative destruction that leads to tumors.

Evidence of Antioxidants' Anticancer Action

The first sign doctors often observe of a potential cancer that is developing in a patient are growths termed *premalignant lesions*. A premalignant lesion consists of tissue that is growing abnormally and have what pathologists call "altered cellular structure." Some of the most common premalignant lesions are colon polyps, oral leukoplakia (white spots on the inside of the mouth), and cervical dysplasia (growth in the uterine cervix). These growths are not cancerous, but, left to themselves, they have a high probability of becoming cancers.

In the case of cervical dysplasia, the premalignant lesion carries a high probability of developing into full-blown cervical cancer. Several population studies have shown that women who consume very little beta-carotene and vitamin C or whose blood contains very little of these antioxidants have increased risk of cervical dysplasia and cervical cancer. One such study revealed that the women who consumed the lowest amount of beta-carotene had double to triple the risk of cervical dysplasia or cervical cancer than the women in the group who consumed the most. When other researchers examined women who had premalignant lesions in this area, their blood levels of beta-carotene were found to be significantly lower than those found in healthy women.

Although beta-carotene can serve as a vitamin A precursor, being converted by the body into vitamin A as needed, apparently its protective action against cervical dysplasia has little to do with its metamorphosis into vitamin A. For when scientists compared the levels of vitamin A in the diets of these women, as compared to beta-carotene, only the beta-carotene seemed to reduce the risk from cervical dysplasia or cancer. As a matter of fact, the vitamin A blood levels were practically the same in the healthy women as in the women with cancerous growths. "These findings suggest that the protective role of beta-carotene is not related solely to its role as a precursor of vitamin A," says Harinder S. Garewal, M.D., Ph.D., associate professor at the University of Arizona and assistant director of the Cancer Prevention and Control Program at the Tucson V. A. Medical Center.

The amount of vitamin C in your diet may also affect your risk of cervical cancer. Researchers have found that a group of women with cervical dysplasia averaged more than 20 percent less vitamin C in the foods they were eating than women without the disease. In these study subjects, the risk of cervical dysplasia for women consuming less than 30 milligrams per day of vitamin C was ten times higher than for women who took in more than 30 milligrams daily. Similarly, comparisons of vitamin C blood levels in other women showed that those suffering from cervical dysplasia had vitamin C levels that averaged less than half the level of healthy women.

Oral Cancer

Every year, thirty thousand people in the United States develop oral cancer. The annual death rate from this disease is close to ten thousand in the United States. Chewing tobacco and drinking alcoholic beverages are two of the major causes of this disease. In parts of the Third World such as New Guinea, Sri Lanka, India, Hong Kong, Taiwan, and sections of South America, high rates of oral cancer are blamed on the custom of chewing betel nuts as well as tobacco and other substances. In those countries about 25 percent of all cancers are found in people's mouths.

Oral cancer is a nasty disease with a couple of insidious characteristics. The illness frequently comes as an evil surprise to many who eschew cigarettes, cigars, or pipes in favor of chewing tobacco, which they mistakenly believe presents a lower health risk. Chewing tobacco may not give you lung cancer, but it significantly increases your risk of developing cancer in your gums, cheeks, and other oral tissues. If you frequently indulge in both alcohol and chewing tobacco, your risk is even greater.

Unfortunately, even when oral cancer is seemingly cured, it is often followed by another episode of cancer somewhere in the upper body. Anywhwere between 10 and 40 percent of those who develop oral cancer will also fall victim to another tumor, usually in the throat. Even if a mouth cancer is caught early and removed, many patients are killed by the second cancer. Doctors blame this secondary outbreak on damage to the epithelial tissue in the throat, which they call field cancerization.

Medical research indicates that a diet high in fruits, vegetables, vitamin A, and beta-carotene or other carotenoids may lower the risk for oral cancer. In a study done in Bombay, India, people who ate vegetables every day had a much lower risk of cancers in the throat and mouth. (Always remember that the vitamins and nutrients in what you eat are as important as the supplements you take.)

Experiments also indicate that beta-carotene and vitamin E are effective against oral cancer. In one experiment, researchers found encouraging results when they tested vitamins on lesions in the mouths of hamsters. (Hamsters were picked because the cancer they get inside their cheeks closely resembles the cancer humans get in their mouths.)

The researchers found that beta-carotene and vitamin E applied to the hamster tumors slowed their growth. When beta-carotene was injected directly into the cancer, the growths decreased even more significantly. These scientists also showed that retinoids—chemicals made from vitamin A—could inhibit the tumors.

In humans, researchers have also investigated the effect of retinoids on precancerous oral lesions, but retinoids in high doses often have strong side effects, including liver and nervous system damage. Researchers also found that after people stopped taking the retinoids, many of the precancerous growths came right back.

Beta-carotene, however, has proven to be a much safer and cheaper treatment. Experiments have shown that beta-carotene by itself or together with vitamin A can cut down on the amount of damaged cells in people at risk for oral cancer.

Beta-Carotene Versus Oral Lesions

In another test in India, researchers gave vitamin A and beta-carotene to people suffering from precancerous lesions. They found that 15 percent of the people taking 180 milligrams of beta-carotene per week for six months had their lesions completely disappear, and more than one out of four of the people taking that much beta-carotene plus 100,000 IU of vitamin A got rid of their growths. At the same time, beta-carotene and vitamin A apparently prevented many new growths from forming.

Stomach Cancer

Do you need vitamin supplements to fight off the carcinogenic effects of your drinking water? It could be, for in many parts of the United States, the drinking water and sometimes the food is filled with nitrates, chemicals that your stomach may convert into cancer-causing substances called nitrosamines. Nitrates, which often run off into the water supply from the irrigation of crops, can be found in especially high amounts in areas of the country where farming is a big business. If you eat a great deal of luncheon meat, which frequently includes nitrates and nitrites (a similar chemical) as preservatives, you may also be getting significant doses.

Not a lot is known about how antioxidant vitamins

interact with cancer-causing chemicals in your stomach, but the evidence that does exist suggests that here, too, taking antioxidant vitamins is probably a smart form of health insurance.

Stomach cancer starts when the lining of the stomach is inflamed, a condition that is called gastritis. The inflammation makes the stomach lining more vulnerable to damage by certain by-products of digestion that linger in your stomach while the food you have eaten interacts with chemicals secreted by the digestive tract.

When a chemical such as one of the nitrosamines is present in someone who has gastritis, the genes within the nucleus of some of the cells that make up the stomach lining can be damaged. This is one of several steps that eventually lead to stomach cancer.

Since lesions that form in the stomach are constantly exposed to the food that flows down the digestive tract, according to Dr. Garewal, it is to be expected that growths in this area are especially sensitive to the carcinogenicity or anticarcinogenicity of anything you swallow.

Research has demonstrated that both vitamins C and E are capable of stopping the stomach from making nitrites and nitrates into nitrosamines. On top of that, studies have shown that taking vitamin C supplements can lower the cancer risk by decreasing the tendency of digestive juices in the stomach to cause genetic mutations.

There are other reasons to take vitamins for your stomach: Studies of gastric juices show that victims of chronic gastritis and atrophic gastritis (a chronic inflammation accompanied by deterioration of the stomach lining) have less vitamin C in their stomachs than healthy people. As a matter of fact, in towns having high rates of stomach cancer deaths and atrophic gastritis, the average blood level of vitamin C has been found to be lower than in towns with fewer stomach problems.

Breathing Easy With Antioxidants

Perhaps no organ in the body is as exposed to pollutants as is the lungs. No matter where you live, chances are there's some kind of industrial chemical floating in the air that you inhale. Chemicals such as carbon monoxide, ozone, and nitrous oxide from factories, car exhaust, and incineration are poured into the atmosphere every hour of the day.

While there is no such thing as total protection from air pollution, recent evidence indicates that the antioxidant vitamins may offset some of its ill effects. Experiments have shown that the airborne pollutants wafting over our streets and avenues damage lungs by means of corrosive free radical reactions that wreak havoc with the little air sacs inside our chests. In theory at least, these reactions can be partially blocked by vitamins C and E (although the only totally effective countermeasure is still a gas mask).

If you are foolish enough to smoke (or unlucky enough to inhale the sidestream smoke from a smoker), that's even more reason to take antioxidants. Cigarette smoke and the other pollutants you are liable to meet can inflame your lungs, stimulating the activity of white blood cells. The commotion among these little protectors of the lungs also produces free radicals that can tear into lung tissue. Animal experiments show that vitamin E may protect us somewhat from these noxious chemicals.

Further supporting the evidence that it would be foolish not to take antioxidant supplements in a polluted society like ours, it has been shown that smokers have less vitamin C in their plasma (the liquid portion of the blood) and in their white blood cells. They also have less vitamin A and carotenes in their plasma. This may be an indication that their nicotine habit is exposing their bodies to enough free radicals to use up a good supply of their antioxidants.

What does this mean for smokers? Certainly, if you smoke and you are at all interested in your further good health, you should kick the habit as soon as possible. If you can't give up cigarettes (or pipes or cigars or whatever it is you are lighting up) you'd be foolish not to take supplements and gulp down as many fruits and vegetables as possible.

Taking supplements is never going to completely offset the negative health effects of smoking, however. Giving up smoking is still the best thing any smoker can do for his or her health.

Summary

Today's polluted environment has led many cancer experts to believe we face an increased risk of cancer. Pesticides in our food, industrial chemicals in our air, increased ultraviolet exposure from the sun due to a depleted radiation-filtering ozone layer, and a high-fat diet are all factors that may be boosting our chances of developing cancer.

Antioxidant vitamins hold out one of the best hopes for forestalling cancer even after its initial stages have taken hold. According to Dr. Garewal, a wide range of experiments with premalignant lesions—growths associated with the development of cancer—demonstrate that certain nutrients can interrupt cancer's progress.

"In experimental animals, vitamins A, C, D, E, B_{12}, riboflavin, and folic acid, as well as choline, calcium, zinc, copper, iron, selenium, and several amino acids have been shown to alter the process of cancer development or carcinogenesis," says Dr. Garewal. In particular,

Dr. Garewal points out, vitamins C and E and beta-carotene may interrupt cancer by means of their anti-oxidant action. "Retinoids [chemicals related to vitamin A] and carotenoids have beneficial effects on cell differentiation, immune function and the interaction of cells with growth factors, all of which may be important in their cancer inhibiting potential," he says. As of yet, the precise means with which they might stop cancer has not been identified.

4

The B Vitamin Complex

B Vitamins

Using the designation *B vitamin complex* for the group of vitamins that are all classified as B vitamins is an old-fashioned, confusing way to name this group of nutrients, but since this is the way these nutrients have traditionally been described, and since they still are denoted this way on vitamin labels, we have to deal with them in this manner.

Why are they all lumped together as a complex? Back in the early days of nutrition research, investigators who were trying to extract micronutrients from food thought they were only going to find two basic kinds: water-soluble and fat-soluble substances.

These researchers, working at the University of Wisconsin just before World War I, named their first discovery *fat-soluble A* and their second *water-soluble B*. Since the term *vitamin* hadn't been invented, they called these chemicals taken out of food *factors*.

Originally, the B factor these scientists thought they had isolated was considered a single substance that prevented the deficiency disease beriberi, but when more lab work was done on this chemical, it was discovered that what had been taken out of food was a group of chemicals that included the chemical that stopped beriberi.

It would have made more sense to give each of these other chemicals completely different names rather than calling them all B vitamins, but other scientists had discovered more food factors and had already assigned these factors alphabet letters. By the time the folks in the lab realized that water-soluble B was in fact a clump of different substances, other folks with notebooks had already designated the chemical that prevents scurvy as water-soluble C, and the nutrient necessary to prevent rickets had been deemed fat-soluble D.

The solution was to keep calling these factors the B factors, while giving each of them their own little subset number. A working definition was that these vitamins were soluble in water and were present in yeast. The factor that prevented beriberi was designated B_1, and the other chemicals received numbers all the way up to B_{17}.

To make things even more confusing, the scientists working on the B factors soon found that some of the substances they had named didn't seem to be important for health at all. Still others had actually been named twice. Obviously, life as a nutrition researcher has never been simple. If you think that the modern-day flow of nutrition discoveries sometimes seems contradictory, rest assured that it's been that way from the beginning.

Anyway, by the time the dust settled on the B factors, B_1, B_2, B_3, B_6, and B_{12} had survived to make it into the textbooks and the rest had been discarded. Eventually, some scientists believe, this outmoded way of talking about this group of vitamins will be eliminated completely, but it doesn't seem likely to happen soon. Even though calling this group of vitamins the B complex is merely a historical artifact, the designation will probably stick for the foreseeable future.

Thiamine (Vitamin B$_1$)

Thiamine's main job in the body is the vital task of assisting conversion of carbohydrates into energy. This vitamin is not stored in the body to any great extent, so you have to consume some every day to avoid a deficiency in it, which will make you very sick, very quickly. Luckily, thiamine occurs in many different foods and extreme deficiency is rare.

Lack of this vitamin used to be common because of dietary peculiarities in some parts of the world. The late nineteenth century investigation of the deficiency disease connected to thiamine, beriberi, was the first scientific study that systematically proved a disease could be caused by the lack of a specific nutrient in the diet. Up until this time, some researchers had shown that types of food could cure diseases such as scurvy, but it was still widely believed that what we now know are diseases caused by nutrient deficiencies were caused by poisons in food.

In the 1880s, Christian Eijkman, a young Dutch doctor, was dispatched by the Dutch government to the East Indies to find a cure for beriberi. This malady was running rampant through parts of Asia where white rice was a dietary mainstay, and it had also struck many parts of South America.

Because of the crucial role thiamine plays in metabolism, the frightening symptoms of beriberi, which occurs when thiamine is completely lacking in the diet, strike swiftly and often lead to a quick death. Victims stop eating and suffer severe mental confusion. Then they may lose feelings in their legs and suffer paralysis, serious heart abnormalities, and breathing problems before dying. In Eijkman's time, young people who appeared healthy would frequently succumb to beriberi with frightening suddenness.

Refined Foods Bring Disease

In Sinhalese, beriberi means weakness. In Japan, the same disease is known as *kakke*. This disease of many names only gained serious proportions in Asia after the industrial revolution reached that continent. Before that time, this condition had only occurred among wealthy Asians.

The reason for the proliferation of beriberi was tied to the spread of the machine age. Before machinery and factories became widespread in the Orient, the rich were the only citizens who could afford to eat polished rice. This food had to be milled intensively by hand or by animal power. The polishing process, which converted the brownish rice to a grain with a sophisticated white gleam, removed the bran that contains the rice's thiamine.

Once steam powered mills began bringing polished rice to the hoi polloi of the Far East, beriberi spread throughout the population. This was one of the first examples of how automated food refining made possible cheap, bland food that jeopardized the nutritional quality of the diets of millions of people.

Chickens Need Thiamine Too

Eijkman's study of the human victims of beriberi left him initially stymied until he noted a similar condition in the poultry residents of the chicken house adjacent to his laboratory. His observations of this disease in animals seemed to hit a dead end when all the birds mysteriously recovered from their disease. Investigating further, he found that during the period of time when the chickens were sick, they had been fed a diet of white, polished rice. When a new employee began feeding the chickens unpolished brown rice whose husks had not been removed (the farmhand thought white rice was too much of a luxury to be fed to birds), the chickens regained their good health.

Eijkman quickly established that he could give chickens the fowl equivalent of beriberi by feeding them polished rice and he could cure the chickens' disease by letting them eat the bran that had been taken off the white rice. Would the same kind of cure work in humans?

Eijkman examined the diet of prison inmates in the Dutch East Indies, and he found that beriberi was hundreds of times more prevalent among prisoners eating polished rice than those on a diet of brown rice. Next he extracted a substance from rice bran that cured and prevented beriberi.

At first, in conformity with the prevailing nutrition theories of the day, Eijkman thought the chemical in the rice bran was an antidote for a poison that was present in white rice. It took almost twenty years for Eijkman and his colleague Gerrit Grijns to grasp the idea that beriberi was caused by a deficiency, not by a toxin. It wasn't until 1907 that the research team announced that rice bran contained a chemical that is necessary to keep people well.

Curing Beriberi at Sea

Curiously enough, a doctor in the Japanese navy had discovered how to cure beriberi even before Eijkman did his work, but his findings seemed to have little effect on what most Asians were eating. In 1884 Kanehiro Takaki experimented with the diets of Japanese sailors in order to understand why they suffered beriberi while British sailors, spending just as much time at sea, remained healthy.

What Takaki found was that the British consumed large amounts of meat and dairy products, but the Japanese mostly ate white rice. Takaki's conclusion was that beriberi was caused by a lack of nitrogen derived from protein. His theory was wrong, but his cure worked. At his urging, the Japanese navy started feeding sailors meat and milk and consequently eliminated beriberi from its ships. Even though it wasn't the nitrogen in these foods that cured the disease, meat and milk contain enough thiamine to prevent deficiency.

Why didn't other Asians, besides Japanese sailors, change their diet? Most Americans also won't change theirs from fatty fast foods that they have been warned may be harmful to their health. Just as Americans are in love with their burgers and fries, Asians were in love with their polished rice. People don't eat healthier foods merely because health experts tell them to. As can be seen time and time again, they'd rather die than give up their dietary habits.

Running Low on Thiamine

Fortunately, in the United States today hardly anyone suffers from beriberi. The only people at risk of severe thiamine deficiency are alcoholics. When you imbibe large amounts of alcohol over an extended period of time, you increase your metabolic need for thiamine but eat fewer foods containing this nutrient. Every time an alcoholic goes to the bathroom, the little thiamine left in the body is excreted.

One reason most of us are safe from thiamine deficiency is because of its presence in white bread, white rice, and many breakfast cereals. Of course, it isn't there naturally, it's there by law. When these foods are refined, all the thiamine is removed. To prevent the possibility of widespread beriberi, U.S. regulations require refiners to fortify white bread and white rice with vitamins, including thiamine.

On those few occasions when beriberi does occur, it is divided into four types: dry beriberi, where victims lose their appetite, lose weight, and lapse into a weary, hopeless mental state; wet beriberi characterized by the buildup of large amounts of fluid in the body (called edema); infantile beriberi, which strikes nursing babies whose mothers are thiamine deficient; and Wernicke-Korsickoff syndrome, which strikes alcoholics. To prevent this condition, some experts have proposed fortifying alcoholic beverages.

Anyone suspected of suffering serious thiamine deficiency should receive competent medical help immediately. These deficiency conditions cause permanent brain damage, and the longer they are left untreated, the more dangerous the outcome.

Get Your Thiamine

Even though overt beriberi is extremely rare and mostly seen among alcoholics, you don't have to be a heavy drinker to increase your need for thiamine. Since this vitamin is used in the metabolism of carbohydrates, those who indulge in intense exercise and those who eat a high carbohydrate diet need extra thiamine, too. That's a good reason to stick to whole grain products such as whole wheat and brown rice. Because the bran is not removed, the thiamine remains in these foods. Of course, white bread and white rice are fortified, but these are still lacking some other nutrients that are not put back in, such as vitamin E and fiber. Brewer's yeast, organ meats such as liver, pork, legumes, and nuts are also good sources of thiamine.

When preparing foods, be aware that thiamine is most often leached out when foods are cooked in water and the water is discarded. For instance, when pasta is boiled, half of the pasta's thiamine ends up in the cooking water and goes down the drain when the pasta is taken off the stove. That probably can't be helped, since there's not much you can do with spaghetti water. However, it is a good reason to not cook your pasta very long and eat it al dente. The shorter the cooking time, the less thiamine is removed.

With other foods, steaming or cooking with a minimum of water and holding down the cooking time will preserve thiamine. Whenever possible, use the cooking water in recipes so that the vitamins in it will be consumed.

Even though it rarely causes thiamine deficiency, be aware that sushi (raw fish) contains enzymes that destroy thiamine. In theory, if your diet consists entirely of polished (unfortified) white rice and raw fish, you could develop thiamine deficiency. But in the United States, most states have laws against selling unfortified white bread and white rice.

Vitamin B$_2$ (Riboflavin)

Riboflavin's basic functions in the human body were not clearly understood by the first vitamin investigators. That is due to the fact that what riboflavin does in the human body is inextricably tied in with the functions of other vitamins. Also, riboflavin deficiency does not show up as a clear-cut, life threatening disease like scurvy or beriberi. That made it still harder for researchers to assign clear-cut functions to riboflavin. Additionally, because of the way riboflavin is distributed in food, if a person is not getting enough of this nutrient, chances are he or she is also deficient in other vitamins, making it harder to isolate the precise signs of riboflavin deficiency.

Consequently, in the early days of vitamin research, investigators mistook symptoms of lack of riboflavin for symptoms of pellagra, the deficiency disease linked to niacin, another B vitamin. It wasn't until the 1930s that riboflavin was adequately understood and scientists discerned its true role in human health.

Riboflavin Helps Make Enzymes

Your body uses riboflavin to shape proteins into enzymes that enable oxygen to get to all the cells in the body. In addition, riboflavin is needed to help vitamin B_6 function properly in its metabolic reactions.

Because riboflavin affects red blood cells, which carry oxygen through the bloodstream, a test of enzymes related to red blood cell activity is sometimes used to calculate a person's riboflavin sufficiency. This measurement, called a test of erythrocyte glutathione reductase (EGR) activity can indicate that the body's riboflavin supply is inadequate before overt signs of deficiency appear. Screening of Americans with tests of EGR activity show that one out of ten of us may not get enough riboflavin.

Experts argue, however, about how harmful a marginal deficiency of riboflavin is to health in the absence of obvious physical signs of riboflavin deficiency, which are not very common. The overt symptoms include cracks at the corner of the mouth, sore throat, burning lips, flaky and inflamed skin, and, if the deficiency is prolonged, victims develop anemia. Usually, alcoholics are at special risk of severe riboflavin deficiency.

Some experts argue that stress and use of birth control pills increase your need for this vitamin although this is not universally accepted. Studies that examined how oral contraceptives affected riboflavin in the body did not come to consistent conclusions.

Still, from all the evidence, it seems like a good idea to at least take the RDA of riboflavin in a multivitamin supplement, particularly if you are a woman who frequently exercises. A study done at Cornell University in Ithaca, New York, in the early 1980s demonstrated that women who work out require more riboflavin than sedentary women. The researchers compared EGR activity in women who jogged with those who rarely exercised and found the joggers needed about 50 percent more of this nutrient.

Other studies have found that those who are lacking riboflavin may suffer depression. Examinations of patients at psychiatric institutions indicated that one out of three have riboflavin deficiency, as well as deficiencies in thiamine and pyridoxine.

Besides getting your riboflavin in a supplement, good dietary sources of this vitamin are meats, fish, poultry, dairy foods, fortified cereals and grains, turnip greens, asparagus, spinach, and broccoli.

Vitamin B$_3$ (Niacin)

The objections some experts make to vitamin supplements are often based on the fact that they are a relatively new form of nutrients. For thousands of years, humans have taken all of their nutrients in food. Nowhere in our culinary history before the twentieth century did anyone take concentrated forms of vitamins, minerals, or any other substance bound up in a pill.

Those who claim that vitamins represent a totally unique twist to human nutrition ignore other sudden substantive changes in our diets. In truth, humans have frequently changed their dietary habits because of technological changes and the discoveries of new foods. Sometimes the results have been beneficial. Other times they are disastrous.

A good lesson in the way changes in nutrition can have unforeseen consequences is demonstrated in the relationship between corn and niacin deficiency. Before Europeans first discovered corn, niacin deficiency was unknown in Europe, but this grain, a dietary staple of the natives of the Western Hemisphere, was eventually responsible for killing thousands of Europeans.

New Food, New Disease

Much has been said about the cultural and physical changes that occurred in both the New World and the Old World after Columbus and other European adventurers opened up the Western Hemisphere to trade (and warfare) with Europe. While these voyages may have resulted in the death by disease of many Native Americans whose immune systems were unprepared for the illnesses introduced to North and South America by the newcomers, the Europeans in their turn suffered serious maladies, too, though theirs were not as catastrophic.

Of the many new foods and agricultural products introduced to Europe as a result of explorations by Columbus and those who came afterward, corn proved to be one of the most popular.

Corn is a nutritious grain, but the type of niacin contained in corn is not readily absorbed by the human body. This was not a problem for Native Americans who prepared corn by first soaking it in lime, a process that converts the food's niacin into a form that is usable by the human digestive tract.

But when the Europeans began eating a diet heavy in corn, they omitted the lime preparation used by Americans. The Europeans who indulged in a diet that was almost exclusively corn often developed pellagra, the devastating deficiency disease caused by niacin deficiency.

The name *pellagra* comes from the Italian term for rough skin, one of the symptoms of this disease. The early signs of pellagra include headaches, weakness in the muscles, stomach problems, diarrhea, and loss of appetite. In severe, prolonged cases, the skin grows rough and cracked and rashes break out on the elbows, knees, and sides of the body. Ulcers appear in the mouth and the tongue grows very red. Eventually, nervous system damage occurs and insanity may result. During the early 1900s, it was found that many patients who were admitted to insane asylums were actually suffering from pellagra.

Similar to most of the other early theories about deficiency diseases, Europeans believed that pellagra was caused by a toxin in corn. To stop the disease, some European countries tried to ban the human consumption of corn altogether. Where the ban succeeded, the disease was eradicated.

In the early history of the United States, not much attention was paid to this deficiency disease, perhaps because most of its victims were the poor and insane. Just before World War I, when the disease became extremely widespread, the government began to spend significant sums to study the high rates of pellagra noted in the Southern states. In 1911 and 1912, separate commissions examined the disease and came to the conclusion that it was caused by a mysterious microbe.

In 1914, Joseph Goldberger, a doctor with the U.S. Public Health Service, found that pellagra could be cured by adding milk, meat, and eggs to the diet.

Goldberger quickly proved his hypothesis by first ridding an orphanage of pellagra by improving the institution's diet and then by giving pellagra to prison inmates by feeding them an incomplete diet.

Still, even though Goldberger presented irrefutable proof of the causes of pellagra, his dietary advice was ignored and the disease continued to ravage many parts of the country, becoming one of the leading causes of death. It was estimated that in the late 1920s there were still around 250,000 cases of pellagra in the United States.

Why did people resist a curative change in diet? Some historians believe that poverty and a laissez-faire attitude on the part of the government was to blame. Pellagra was a disease of the poor and no one cared enough about it to spend the funds to wipe it out at that time.

Dog Disease Yields Niacin

Even after it was discovered that certain foods caused pellagra, it was laboratory work on dogs that allowed scientists to isolate and synthesize niacin, the specific vitamin related to this deficiency disease. In canines, niacin deficiency disease is called black tongue, a condition in which dogs' tongues actually turn dark blue and they suffer diarrhea and oral ulcers. Carefully manipulating the diets of these animals, Goldberger worked for almost ten years to find what he called *factor P-P,* the pellagra preventive factor. Soon it became known as vitamin B_2, though for a while it was known as vitamin G, in honor of Dr. Goldberger's work.

What confused the early work on niacin and still confuses many people about this vitamin today is that you don't always have to consume it in your food to have a sufficient supply in your body. You can make this vitamin out of tryptophan, an amino acid contained in foods like milk and beef. When the scientists finally felt secure in their synthesis of the anti-pellagra factor, which they wanted to call vitamin B_3, they found that it was the same substance as nicotinic acid, a compound that had first been identified in the 1890s.

In the late 1930s, when the government was finally ready to fortify foods with this pellagra-preventive nutrient, officials found themselves with a public relations problem. Because the name nicotinic acid is similar to nicotine, the drug contained in tobacco, it was popularly believed that food was about to be fortified with tobacco. Thus the name niacin was invented to replace nicotinic acid and dispel public concern.

Different Forms of Vitamin B_3

When trying to determine how much niacin you get in your diet, you must keep in mind that many of the protein foods you eat probably contain tryptophan, the amino acid your body can make into niacin. For instance, the tryptophan in a cup of milk can be converted into the equivalent of about half of your requirement of niacin. You won't find this information on the food label. When niacin is listed on labels, only the niacin actually found in the food is included. The niacin your body might make from the tryptophan in the food is ignored.

As with many of the other water-soluble vitamins, niacin is lost when foods are boiled and the cooking water is discarded. If you reuse the cooking water in other recipes, you can save some of the niacin. Most whole grains, with the exception of corn, are good niacin sources. Your body doesn't store much niacin, so you should eat some every day. It is a fairly stable vitamin, so when foods are stored their niacin content usually decreases very slowly.

If you take vitamin supplements, another point to keep in mind is that niacin supplements are also sold in the form of nicotinamide which, as far as its action in the body is concerned, is the equivalent of niacin. The difference is that when you take very large amounts of this form of the vitamin, nicotinamide does not cause the flushing (vascular dilation) that results when you take big doses of niacin or nicotinic acid.

Niacin and Cholesterol

In the 1950s it was discovered that taking large doses of niacin lowers triglycerides, a form of fat found in the blood that is believed to be a risk factor for heart disease. To have this effect, however, the vitamin has to be taken as nicotinic acid in very large doses—between 3 and 9 grams a day. Aside from the unpleasant feelings this dosage can produce—you turn red and flushed, and momentarily feel uncomfortably hot—doses this high can be hard on your liver.

Therefore, you should never take large doses of nicotinic acid without close supervision by a doctor. When you consistently ingest this substance, you need to have frequent blood tests to make sure your liver function is adequate. In some people, large doses of nicotinic acid may cause liver damage and they have to discontinue it. Taken in these amounts, nicotinic acid ceases to act as a vitamin and is considered a very powerful drug.

Vitamin B$_6$

New discoveries in the field of nutrition often seem to contradict each other. That's why people often complain that they cannot count on nutrition researchers to give them dependable advice on the healthiest foods to eat or the best vitamins to take. The constantly evolving science of nutrition seems to leap ahead with new revelations, only to constantly backtrack with contrary advice. Today's front page headline, "Stop Eating the Saturated Fat in Butter, Switch to Margarine!" too often becomes tomorrow's back page retraction: "Hydrogenated Oils in Margarine Linked to Heart Disease!"

A brief look at the history of vitamin B_6 shows why it is so difficult for scientific investigators to come up with definitive findings on the long-range effects of nutrients on our health. Much of modern nutrition research is performed on animals, since it is considered unethical to experiment on humans. Many people object to experimentation on animals as well. Even when animal experiments point to particular functions of nutrients, these findings do not always yield results applicable to people.

For instance, it has been shown that some animals live much longer if they eat less food. This has led to the call by some researchers for people to eat less and live longer. Unfortunately, there has never been a shred of evidence in research performed on humans to show that this principle applies to people.

The same kind of difficulty with using animals to test the functions of nutrients led to complications in understanding the role and identity of vitamin B_6. Originally, rats were used in attempts to understand what deficiencies this vitamin might cause. Scientists thought that a skin condition in rats caused by vitamin B_6 deficiency was linked to pellagra in humans.

It wasn't. Pellagra is caused by a deficiency of niacin. The rat skin condition was caused by a cluster of three different chemicals that rats and, as it turned out, humans, make into the same coenzyme.

What is still called vitamin B_6 is actually three different chemicals that all behave similarly when you take them in your food or vitamin pills. The nutrients, pyridoxine, pyridoxal, and pyridoxamine, all help with processing protein in the body.

Dangers of B_6 Deficiency

The fact that the vitamin B_6 compounds are necessary for more than five dozen different protein-related reactions in the body make this vitamin vital for good health. Early in the investigation of this vitamin it was found that some people who seemed to be suffering from pellagra (niacin deficiency) did not recover when given niacin, riboflavin, or thiamine, but did get better when administered B_6.

Still, it was unclear exactly what pure B_6 deficiency looked like since so many foods contain a form of this vitamin. Perhaps out of frustration, researchers during and after World War II tried to decipher B_6's functions, got a little carried away, and performed experiments that took some bizarre twists. In the 1940s, a Canadian investigator named W. W. Hawkins induced B_6 deficiency in himself by going on a diet that totally lacked B_6. After two months on the diet, he lost weight, suffered anemia, his blood pressure fell, and he became depressed and confused, but not so confused that he didn't remember to start eating foods containing B_6 so as to recover from his deficiency.

In another study—this one a bit more distasteful—doctors at the New York University School of Medicine induced B_6 deficiency in two "mentally defective" infants. One infant developed convulsions. Both babies failed to gain weight. The results of this test showed that B_6 is necessary for normal growth in babies and essential for normal red blood cells and brain function.

How's Your Vitamin B_6 Status?

Whether or not Americans receive enough vitamin B_6 in their diets is another source of controversy. One of the few clear-cut instances of widespread B_6 deficiency occurred in the 1950s when babies being fed an infant formula began to suffer mysterious convulsions. It turned out that the company preparing the formula had cooked it at higher temperatures than normal to kill bacteria. This high temperature had not only sterilized the formula, it had also destroyed the food's B_6. When the babies were put on formula containing B_6, they recovered.

Except for rare instances like that, pure B_6 deficiency seems to be rare. Usually, to be seriously deficient in this vitamin, you need to be eating so little that you will be suffering general malnutrition, but many people may be marginally deficient in vitamin B_6.

An investigation in Texas found that only one woman out of the seventy-four taking part in the study was getting the RDA of this vitamin (currently the RDA for women is 1.6 milligrams per day). Another study performed in Florida showed that pregnant women were generally only consuming half their RDA (2.2 milligrams for pregnant women). The vitamin is important: The babies born to mothers who consumed adequate B_6 were healthier than the other newborns.

Consequently, many experts feel that pregnant women, or those who plan to become pregnant soon, should take moderate supplements of B_6 (usually sold in the form of pyridoxine) in the amounts of about 6 to 8 milligrams a day. Often this can be found in a multivitamin.

B_6 Versus PMS and Morning Sickness

Over the years, many people have advocated vitamin B_6 as a treatment for premenstrual syndrome (PMS), although the evidence for this is debatable. In a study of the vitamin's effects on PMS, a group of more than 600 women were given either placebos (sugar pills) or pyridoxine and then, through three menstrual cycles, were evaluated for PMS symptoms such as bloating, depression, irritability, and headache. Almost three-quarters of the women in the study noted a decrease in some symptoms whether or not they were taking the placebo or the actual vitamin. Overall, however, the women taking the vitamin felt slightly better—but only slightly—than the placebo group.

This means that it is safe to try pyridoxine supplementation for PMS, but don't expect miracles. For this purpose, it is probably not a good idea to take more than a daily 10-milligram supplement.

For many years, pregnant women have taken Bendectin, a medicine for morning sickness that includes pyridoxine as well as other medicine. Is the B_6 in this medication effective against this problem? A test of pregnant women that compared a placebo to B_6 showed virtually no difference between the two. Still, Bendectin seems to help some women. (On the other hand, during pregnancy, morning sickness usually goes away on its own after a while, anyway.)

Carpal Tunnel Syndrome

Researchers have also investigated whether or not pyridoxine supplements can alleviate carpal tunnel syndrome, a nerve problem in the arm and hands caused by repetitive motion such as typing at a keyboard day after day for long hours. The syndrome is caused by pressure on a nerve that goes into the wrist. At its worst, the affliction causes virtual paralysis of the hand and makes any movement of the thumb or wrist extremely painful.

Surgically, carpal tunnel syndrome is treated by cutting into the arm and relieving the pressure on the nerve, but in some studies, supplements of up to 300 milligrams of pyridoxine daily were found to relieve the syndrome. However, still other studies find that pyridoxine does not always bring relief.

If you decide to take these kinds of supplements, it's best to be under a doctor's supervision. Some people have suffered neurological problems and trouble walking from taking large, continuous supplements of pyridoxine. In one well-known report from the Albert Einstein School of Medicine in New York, it was found that persons taking from 500 to 6,000 milligrams of pyridoxine a day lost feeling in their extremities and had difficulty standing and walking. Some of these people had taken large supplements for only two months, others for more than three years.

In another case, more than one hundred women at a private clinic had been given an average of about 120 milligrams of pyridoxine to treat PMS, depression, and other problems. These women suffered bone pain, numbness in their hands and feet, muscle weakness, and some had to use a cane in order to walk. After stopping the vitamin, it took some of the women up to six months to recover from their neurological complications, though most recovered after about three months.

Animal studies show that this vitamin may help keep the immune system working properly, so there may be evidence that taking small doses of B_6 at or close to the RDA is beneficial. Animals deprived of B_6 display symptoms of immune systems that don't function well. Other animal studies seem to show that B_6 deficiency may encourage certain types of cancers. It is thought that since B_6 is needed at crucial stages when each cell's DNA is being reproduced, lack of this nutrient may cause cell division to go awry, leading to possible tumors.

Still, despite the fact that some experts think we are almost all a little deficient in B_6, if you take supplements, don't overdo it. This is one vitamin where a daily dose of close to the RDA (2.2 milligrams) should be plenty for those who want to be sure they are getting enough. More than that is probably unnecessary; much more than that may give you problems.

And even though your body makes B_6 from the amino acid tryptophan, you should never take tryptophan supplements. Several years ago, all tryptophan supplements were supposed to have been recalled when some people taking these supplements died from a blood disease linked to the supplements. Even now, years later, no one has been able to figure out if it was the tryptophan that killed these supplement takers or a contaminant that somehow got into their pills. To play it safe, never take a tryptophan supplement.

Vitamin B_{12}

Vitamin B_{12} has traditionally had a reputation as an energy booster. For years, doctors have given injections of B_{12} along with other substances to give their patients feelings of well-being and euphoria. However, it has been revealed that many of these vitamin-dispensing physicians also included amphetamines in the injections. This explains the euphoria. Despite the claims that vitamin B_{12} will boost your spirits, there is little or no evidence that under most circumstances this nutrient will give you a lift.

The most serious problem for those suffering a significant lack of vitamin B_{12} is pernicious anemia, a type of anemia that acquired its intimidating name due to its deadly nature. Untreated, this condition is often fatal. Although no one before the twentieth century realized that pernicious anemia was connected to a nutrient deficiency, it was recognized in the 1800s that those suffering this disease did have some kind of problem with their digestion.

In the early 1900s, researchers began to look for a dietary cause for pernicious anemia. The first solid clue as to which nutrient could cure this condition came from research with anemic dogs. Studies showed that these canines would recover somewhat from their anemia when fed liver. Consequently, it was found that many anemic humans would also improve when fed liver. Although the recovery of the dogs pointed the way to the discovery of vitamin B_{12}, later researchers found that it was actually the iron in the liver, not the food's B_{12} content that improved the health of these anemic animals.

Even with the knowledge of which foods could usually relieve pernicious anemia, medical researchers were disappointed to find that not all anemia patients recovered when fed the appropriate diet. These unfortunates had digestive systems that refused to absorb the factor, later confirmed as B_{12}, which was present in the liver and also in beef, eggs, and many red meats.

Interestingly enough, many bacteria can make their own vitamin B_{12}, but it was by experimenting on a bacterium that needed to consume this nutrient from liver in order to survive that researchers at one of the big drug companies finally isolated what they named vitamin B_{12}. Again, even after this chemical was synthesized, not all victims of pernicious anemia responded to treatment with this vitamin. Their digestive tracts were incapable of absorbing it. For these anemia victims, injections of small amounts of this nutrient, a technique that bypasses the digestive tract by introducing the nutrient right into the blood, proved to be sufficient to restore good health.

Some people can't absorb B_{12} because this vitamin has to combine with another protein in the stomach before the nutrient can pass through the walls of the digestive tract. It is the combination of this protein secreted by the stomach and vitamin B_{12} that has to be absorbed. B_{12} alone passes undigested out of the body. Those who need vitamin B_{12} injections have stomachs that are unable to produce this helpful protein.

Sources of Vitamin B_{12}

Ironically, while many bacteria are capable of making vitamin B_{12}, it is only the foods of animal origin in the human diet that contain significant amounts of this nutrient. In other words, to get this vitamin from the things we eat, we have to consume animals that eat these bacteria and store the vitamin in their flesh. Then we humans, at the top of the food chain, take in the vitamin in the hamburgers on our buns and the meat on our dinner plates.

This leaves vegetarians devoid of this vitamin unless they take supplements or they include milk or eggs in their diet. Fortunately, healthy adults, whether vegetarians or omnivores, need very little B_{12} to maintain their health. It is estimated that if you were a carnivore yesterday but became a vegetarian tomorrow and stopped consuming all foods containing vitamin B_{12}, it might take you up to a decade to use up all of the vitamin B_{12} stashed away in your body. Many studies indicate it often takes about three years for half of your stored B_{12} to be excreted.

However, since vegetarian foods generally lack B_{12}, vegetarians should take a supplement containing the RDA for this vitamin: 2 micrograms a day for adults. If you are an omnivore who consumes your share of meat and plan to live a long time, you may also be justified in taking a small supplement. Studies show that after age sixty, your levels of B_{12} decline, although whether or not they decline enough to compromise your health is arguable. In any case, building up your stores of this vitamin before you reach senior citizenship may help keep your body's supply adequate.

Pregnant and Nursing Mothers

There are two other important occasions that usually necessitate taking B_{12} supplements: pregnancy and nursing. Despite the body's tendency to hold on to this vitamin for long periods of time, pregnant and nursing mothers who are vegetarians almost always should take this vitamin. There has been at least one report of a vegetarian nursing mother—who remained in good health herself—whose infant suffered from serious B_{12} deficiency. In that case, the baby was apparently doing well for the first few months of life, only to lapse into a comatose state at about six months of age. When blood tests showed he was suffering from severe anemia, B_{12} injections helped him return to normalcy.

The mother of this infant was in her twenties and had not eaten any foods of animal origin for almost ten years at the time she became pregnant. Even though the B_{12} level in her blood proved to be within what was considered a normal range and she was not anemic, her breast milk, the baby's main source of nutrition, contained only a miniscule amount of this nutrient.

Although this kind of serious B_{12} deficiency is relatively rare, pregnant and nursing mothers who are strict vegetarians are advised to take a supplement containing the RDA for vitamin B_{12}, which is 2.6 micrograms a day. As a matter of fact, to be on the safe side, experts advise all pregnant and nursing mothers, even if they are carnivores, to take a multivitamin containing the RDA of B_{12} and to consult their doctors about their nutritional needs. Infants should receive a multivitamin supplement with the RDA for infants, which is 0.3 micrograms a day.

Folate

While being a vegetarian may limit the amount of vitamin B_{12} you consume in your diet, eating vegetarian foods has the opposite relationship to folate. Most vegetarians should have no problem consuming this vitamin, which is found in good supply in leafy green vegetables such as broccoli, spinach, kale, and asparagus as well as in wheat. On the other hand, Americans who studiously avoid fruits and vegetables in favor of fast food fare (You know who you are!) may be chronically short of this important nutrient. In addition, those who overindulge in alcohol may also run short of folate.

Despite its importance for human health, folate or folic acid (actually a group of about 100 active forms of this nutrient) doesn't seem to get the publicity given to more well-known vitamins such as vitamin C or beta-carotene. As a result, most people don't know about this vitamin or they misunderstand it. Although we do not need too much of this vitamin, the little bit that is necessary is crucial for the formation of red blood cells and the reproduction of DNA throughout the body.

Folic Acid's Complicated Role in the Body

Because of its interaction with vitamin B_{12} in many processes in the body, folic acid has been a misunderstood vitamin ever since the first nutrition researchers began to look for it. After vitamin B_{12} extract from liver was found to relieve many cases of anemia, it was discovered that, as the extract was made purer and purer (containing more and more B_{12} and less and less of other nutrients), some patients were not helped by it. They enjoyed better health when treated with a less pure extract.

That made it evident that there was something else in liver besides B_{12} that was necessary to avoid anemia. Eventually, in the 1940s, using about eight thousand pounds of spinach as their starting material, researchers at the University of Texas extracted a chemical they called folic acid or folate. This name is taken from the Latin for leaf: *folium*. The formal chemical name for the forms of this vitamin is pteroylglutamic acid, abbreviated as PGA.

Soon after its synthesis, folate was the treatment of choice for anemic patients. This proved to be a mistake. Both vitamin B_{12} and folate must be present in the diet for folate to be usable in our bodies. Doctors found that liver extracts, which contain both nutrients, worked better for anemia than did pure folate.

Folate Helps Make New Cells

Since folate's role in the body is tied in with vitamin B_{12}, when you run short of folate, you are usually deficient in other vitamins as well. That's why there are few cases of folate deficiency occuring all by itself without the presence of other deficiencies. In one case where a researcher purposely fed himself a diet short of folate, he suffered insomnia, forgetfulness, and irritability. Then, after about twenty weeks of a diet deficient in this nutrient, he developed anemia. At that point he began taking folate supplements.

To make himself folate deficient, this researcher boiled all of his food and discarded the water, an action that destroyed or eliminated most of the water-soluble vitamins, including all of the B vitamins, folic acid, pantothenic acid, biotin, and vitamin C. He then supplemented himself with all of the water-soluble vitamins except folate. This method of destroying water-soluble vitamins in the lab presents an important lesson for cooks at home. To preserve these nutrients, use as little water as possible when preparing food. If possible, when boiling foods, use the cooking water in an appropriate recipe. Much of the vitamins from your food will be in that water. The National Research Council, which oversees the RDAs, estimates that during household preparation of food, as much as 50 percent of the folate in food may be destroyed.

Since folate is important for the proper development of new cells, the most important time to take supplements with this nutrient is if you are pregnant, trying to become pregnant, or nursing a newborn. Without sufficient folate, newborns and their mothers may suffer anemia. Pregnant women deficient in folate are subject to greater risk of miscarriage and serious bleeding problems.

Folate and Birth Defects

Most recently, it has also been shown that babies born to mothers who lack sufficient folate run a greater risk of birth defects. In particular, conditions known as neural tube defects seem to occur more frequently in women who don't get enough of this nutrient.

Spina bifida and anencephaly, two types of neural tube defects, are presently the most common birth defects in the United States as well as in other countries. These problems in the developing fetus occur when the brain and the spine of the embryo fail to close correctly. In spina bifida, a gap is left in the protective sheath supposed to cover the spinal cord. In anencephaly, the brain is partially or completely missing.

Studies in five European countries as well as Israel and Canada demonstrated a more than 70 percent decrease in the risk of these birth defects when pregnant women were given 4 milligrams of folate a day. In this double-blind study, scientists gave either vitamins or placebos to pregnant women who had already given birth to one baby with a neural tube defect. These women are at increased risk of having a second baby with the defect. During the research, the risk of birth defects in children of women not given the vitamin was seen to be so great, that the study was cut short.

Unfortunately, when it comes to getting enough folate, there's plenty of evidence that a lot of Americans are just not eating enough fresh vegetables, the major source of the nutrient. A large-scale survey of what Americans are eating showed that more than one out of six women between the ages of twenty and forty-four years of age don't eat enough folate-rich foods. Among adolescents in lower income groups, it was estimated that about 50 percent may be deficient.

These widespread deficiencies may also be putting women and smokers at risk for cancer. Research at the University of Alabama revealed that women with cervical dysplasia, precancerous lesions that often develop into cervical cancer, and smokers with precancerous tissue in their lungs both had low levels of folate.

In these diseases, researchers theorize that the premalignant developments may at least partially be due to folate deficiency that allows cells' genetic material to reproduce incorrectly. For women, a sexually transmitted virus sets the events in motion that cause cervical dysplasia. Healthy cervical cells with sufficient folate may be able to mitigate the virus's effects, but a lack of folate may make the viral infection more carcinogenic and likely to result in cervical cancer, the ninth most common cause of cancer death in women in the United States.

In the smokers, the researchers believe that vitamin supplements with folate and B_{12} might be able to reduce the severity of precancerous developments in the lungs. In several studies, they produced indications of beneficial health effects when they gave smokers 25 times the RDA for folic acid, which is 10 milligrams, and 167 times the RDA for B_{12}, which is 0.5 milligrams. They also used a special kind of B_{12} for the special purposes of their study.

These researchers caution that smokers should not assume that they can lower their risk of lung cancer by taking vitamins. For one thing, lung cancer is only one disease that smoking causes. It also causes heart disease, emphysema, and other kinds of cancer. It makes you ugly by causing wrinkles, too. The only way to cut the risk of smoking, they emphasize, is to stop smoking.

They also caution that their research should not be used as a rationale for anyone to take vitamin supplements. However, it seems as though reasonable people might conclude that their findings show the usefulness of eating a healthy diet full of fresh fruits and vitamins and at least considering the possibility of taking supplements that supply the RDA for vitamins B_{12} and folate. Even if you are not a smoker, you probably inhale polluted air much of the time, and almost all of us occasionally inhale a smoker's sidestream smoke. In these civilized circumstances, a little vitamin defense is probably a prudent idea.

A few cautions about folate: Since this nutrient interacts with vitamin B_{12} in complicated ways, taking large doses of folate might theoretically mask a case of pernicious anemia in some people. In other words, if you took megadoses of folate and you unknowingly suffered pernicious anemia, a blood test would not indicate this problem, but you might suffer neurological damage before your anemia could be diagnosed.

Another potential problem can arise if you suffer epilepsy or take anticonvulsant drugs for any reason. Folate can defeat the effectiveness of these medications. Also, some doctors have been using anti-folate drugs to treat certain kinds of cancer, psoriasis, arthritis, and a host of other diseases. It is thought that while folic acid may stop precancerous growths, it is possible that a folate deficiency may kill cancerous tumors that are already established. If you are being treated with such a drug, you probably should not be taking a folate supplement. If you are taking any drugs at all, you should consult with your doctor before taking vitamin supplements.

A problem you probably don't have to worry about is zinc. Nutrition scientists used to believe that folate supplements interfered with the body's zinc absorption. This has been shown to be true in laboratory animals that were fed very large amounts of folate, but if you keep your daily folate supplementation down to between 5 and 15 milligrams a day, experts do not believe that this should be a problem.

Pantothenic Acid

A close look at the vitamins humans need to stay healthy displays effects and interactions similar to a construction of twisting mazes. Follow the metabolic pathway down which a vitamin travels, acting as a coenzyme that takes part in a multitude of processes, and soon you will cross the paths traveled by other vitamins. These pathways in the life-preserving processes of your body intersect countless times. As a result, it is often difficult to isolate the result of a single vitamin deficiency. More often, deficiencies occur in groups. Vitamins work cooperatively, a fact that obscures an individual vitamin's particular function. That complicates the scientist's job of deciphering our requirements for these nutrients or predicting the result of being deficient in a single vitamin.

Because the functions of pantothenic acid, one of the B vitamins, is so interwoven with the functions of other vitamins, scientists have had a tough time pinpointing exactly what a deficiency of this vitamin alone should look like in humans. In the early 1930s, pantothenic acid was identified as a nutrient that yeast needed to survive. Later in that decade researchers found that what they thought was a form of chicken pellagra (which would have been caused by a niacin deficiency) was actually a poultry skin ailment caused by a lack of pantothenic acid.

Studies in rats just before World War II showed that pantothenic acid kept rat fur from turning gray (a condition known as achromotrichia), helped the rat's reproductive organs function properly, and was necessary for the health of rats' adrenal glands. In humans, this vitamin is also important for two of these three functions: It preserves the health of your adrenal glands, and it aids in the production of sex hormones. Unfortunately, despite the claims by some health "experts," this vitamin, even when taken in megadoses, will do nothing for gray hair.

As was the case in the early research of many of the other vitamins, evidence of this nutrient's deficiency in people came from populations in Asia that subsisted on unfortified, polished white rice. In this case, the population in question were Allied prisoners of war held by the Japanese during World War II. Fed a very meager diet that contained little besides polished rice, these soldiers suffered a wide range of vitamin deficiencies including pellagra and beriberi.

In addition to the deficiency symptoms familiar to doctors, many of these prisoners also suffered from an intense burning feeling in their feet. This peculiar sensation seemed to subside during the day but was torturous throughout the night. Prisoners kept their feet in buckets of water for hours, or walked barefoot on the cold ground to stop the agony. In the winters, many lost toes and feet to frostbite because of their inability to keep their feet covered while suffering this burning feeling.

When these prisoners were treated with niacin and thiamine to clear up the pellagra and beriberi that many of them also suffered, the burning sensations persisted. A researcher working in India, Dr. Corish Gopalan, found that pantothenic acid relieved the burning foot sensation when other B vitamins failed.

It wasn't until after the war that an isolated pantothenic acid deficiency in humans—without deficiency of other vitamins—was demonstrated. Even then, in research reported in 1959, feeding prisoners at a jail in Iowa a diet lacking in pantothenic acid wasn't enough to produce an obvious deficiency. Researchers had to give these volunteers a drug called methylpantothenic acid that stopped the action of this nutrient in the body. Then and only then did signs of pantothenic acid deficiency clearly show up. More recently, scientists were able to reproduce the deficiency by giving subjects a semisynthetic diet.

In these studies, the pure deficiency of this nutrient made the subjects feel listless and tired. They also complained of stomachaches and irritability. Some complained of the burning feet the POWs had reported.

In the real world, the world in which you and I dine on fast food, indulge in snacks at the movies, and have so much trouble eating just one potato chip, pure pantothenic acid deficiency hardly ever happens, if it ever happens at all. Part of the reason is that the nutrient appears in a vast variety of foods. It is abundant in meat, legumes (peanuts, lentils, beans), and whole grains. There is also some pantothenic acid in fruits, vegetables, and milk. Some is also made by the bacteria in your intestine, although no one has been able to figure out if that source enters your body or is merely eliminated in the bathroom.

The ubiquitous nature of pantothenic acid means that no one is sure how much you need. All they've been able to figure out is about how much you eat. The

National Research Council (NRC), the folks who bring us the RDAs, haven't computed an RDA for pantothenic acid. Quoting studies that show we all eat about 5 to 10 milligrams a day of this nutrient, the NRC has figured out what it calls "estimated safe and adequate daily dietary intakes" of this nutrient. They figure that adult servings of 4 to 7 milligrams a day of pantothenic acid "should be safe and adequate."

As for pregnant and nursing women, the NRC reports never hearing of a pantothenic acid deficiency in mothers or their babies. It does point out that a lot of pantothenic acid ends up in mother's milk. That leads the council to figure that mothers and mothers-to-be can get by on the same pantothenic acid that everybody else is eating in their food. Since there's so much pantothenic acid in human milk, the council also speculates that nursing mothers get a pantothenic supplement from the bacteria in their intestines.

Where does that leave anyone who is thinking about taking pantothenic acid in their vitamin supplements? The stuff, according to all reports, is notoriously nontoxic, although there have been reports that people taking doses of 10 to 20 grams every day suffered some diarrhea and retained water, but people taking 10 grams a day for six weeks suffered no ill effects.

Will extra pantothenic acid be of benefit? There is little evidence that megadoses of this nutrient will improve your health. In the past, some vitamin marketers have claimed that pantothenic acid will make your gray hair darker, but there is no evidence that it has any effect on hair, even though it makes rat fur less gray. Some vitamin outlets claimed it was good for sore feet, too. But unless you are eating the kind of limited diet fed to malnourished prisoners of war or subjects in a controlled study, it is doubtful that your foot problems have anything to do with a pantothenic acid deficiency. While pantothenic acid is involved in a wide variety of metabolic functions, this is one vitamin that does not seem to cry out for you to take it as a supplement.

Biotin

Want to know how hard it is to be biotin deficient? It takes careful planning, or an extreme fondness for raw egg whites. For, while this sulfur-containing vitamin is found in so many different foods, including egg yolks, that it's tough to run short, there is a chemical in raw egg whites that blocks your biotin metabolism. There is also the occasional person who has a genetic defect that also impairs biotin metabolism.

For most of us, biotin is the kind of quirky nutrient that a deranged nutritionist might have dreamed up to teach us a lesson in why we should eat balanced meals and stay away from unusual diets that emphasize one particular food. As an example, one of the few cases on record of someone suffering biotin deficiency involves a fanatic raw egg aficionado, a Boston resident, who was so devoted to his raw egg habit that he moved out of his house (deserting his family) so he could live on his own chicken farm. On his farm he had enough chickens to feed his obsession with anywhere from two to ten raw eggs a day, which he accompanied with up to four quarts of wine per diem. Why he didn't move to a winery, is not explained in the medical report.

This wine and egg maven was soon suffering from a variety of symptoms such as persistent scaly skin, nausea, loss of appetite, and depression. It was a full-blown biotin deficiency. Oh, yes, his cholesterol probably went up, too. For that is another symptom. When he kicked the raw egg habit, he recovered.

Vitamin H

In the early days of biotin research, it was proposed that this nutrient be called vitamin H. Researchers found that if they fed rats a diet that mostly consisted of raw egg whites, their skin and hair suffered, and then they died. Vitamin H was the substance that seemed to prevent this deficiency disease. Another way of saving the animals' lives was to feed them cooked egg white since cooking changes the avidin so that it does not bind up biotin and make it unusable.

In a later study, four people were fed a biotin-deficient diet along with the requisite raw egg whites, and after about three months they were found to have the expected dry and scaly skin. These subjects also grew depressed, lethargic, and anxious. Finally, when they grew anorectic and refused to eat, the researchers fed them daily supplements of biotin and they quickly regained their appetites and their health.

The occurrence of biotin deficiency in the everyday world outside of a medical setting is a rare event. It mostly troubles the rare infant born with a genetic inability to use biotin. It occasionally may arise in hospital patients fed intravenously with a nutrient solution that omits biotin. For normal adults, biotin can be had in liver, egg yolk (cook those eggs!), soy, cereals, and yeast.

Just remember to stay off the raw egg whites.

5

Vitamin C

It seems like at least half of all nutrition experts argue about vitamin C at least half of the time. Besides being a nutrient, vitamin C has served as a kind of nutritive football tossed around by dietitians, nutrition scientists, the National Research Council, the vitamin companies, and health writers. At the head of the list of those who are on the side for the benefits of this nutrient is Dr. Linus Pauling, Nobel prize winner and designated quarterback of the vitamin C controversy. With the publication of his book *Vitamin C and the Common Cold* back in 1970, Dr. Pauling started the endless media blitz surrounding vitamin C by claiming that taking large doses of this nutrient could reduce the risk of catching a cold.

More than twenty years later, Dr. Pauling, who is now in his nineties, is still taking massive amounts of vitamin C (along with other vitamins) and still raising a ruckus by claiming wondrous powers for vitamin C. Many establishment medical people think he's overstating the case for this nutrient, although they grudgingly concede the vitamin does more than they used to acknowledge.

Study by study, the medical evidence of the health benefits of vitamin C has been building. Research now shows that as an antioxidant vitamin, in conjunction with other antioxidants like vitamin E and beta-carotene, vitamin C apparently does a heroic job of protecting our bodies from the damage of oxidants. In some circumstances, vitamin C may even spare the other antioxidants in our body from harm and preserve their power.

The Structure of Vitamin C

The lack of this vitamin causes a clear-cut deficiency disease called scurvy. Today, according to the National Research Council, the only Americans at serious risk of developing scurvy are infants fed entirely on cow's milk or senior citizens who are eating a very limited diet.

However, as noted on page 22, scurvy used to be a widespread problem, especially among sailors on long ocean voyages. Since the best dietary sources of vitamin C are fresh fruits and vegetables, crews on ships that were stocked only with preserved meats and grains ran a high risk of this deficiency disease. On some long voyages, more than half the sailors succumbed to scurvy.

Scurvy is an ugly disease. Vitamin C is necessary for the synthesis of collagen, a protein that forms the basic fiber that holds our teeth in our gums, reinforces the skin, strengthens the blood vessels, keeps the bones strong, and cements organs together. The structure of the capillaries depends on collagen, as does the proper formation of connective tissue. Stop consuming vitamin C for an extended period of time, and your teeth fall out, blood pools in hemorrhages under the skin, your gums swell and bleed, bones break easily, and your skin becomes uncomfortably dry.

Like a painful special effect in a sci-fi movie, scurvy makes your entire body fall apart as the intercellular cement holding all your organs together fails to work. Given the grisly stages this disease goes through, it must have been truly frightening to have been aboard a ship at sea when much of the crew succumbed to this deficiency.

By the 1600s, many sailors knew the key to preventing scurvy was fresh fruits and vegetables. Certainly, natives of North America had demonstrated to Jacques Cartier that a tea made of spruce needles (containing vitamin C) could cure scurvy. Other captains of the period have left written records noting the usefulness of lemons and produce. European society, stuck in its dietary habits, however, refused to officially acknowledge prevention methods for this scourge until the 1790s when rules were drawn up requiring sailors to receive rations of lemon juice.

Few Animals Need Vitamin C

Interestingly enough, humans are one of the very few species that need to consume vitamin C in the diet. Most other animals can make this vitamin for themselves. Only guinea pigs, primates (apes, monkeys, and gorillas), the Indian fruit eating bat, a variety of Persian songbird, and a very few other animals need to eat this nutrient.

When early researchers fed a restricted diet of polished rice to guinea pigs in the hope of eliciting the symptoms of beriberi (a thiamine deficiency), they instead produced the guinea pig equivalent of scurvy. When other researchers tried to produce scurvy in rats, nothing happened. What they didn't know was that rats cannot develop scurvy; their bodies manufacture all the vitamin C they need for good health.

Finally, it was found that the antiscorbutic or scurvy-preventing factor that cured the guinea pigs also worked on human scurvy. An enterprising chemist named Albert

Szent-Györgyi demonstrated that the identical anti-scurvy chemical was contained in cabbage, lemon juice, and human glands. It was named ascorbic acid, the acid that prevents scurvy.

Do We All Suffer From Vitamin C Deficiency?

By a kind of roundabout logic, Dr. Linus Pauling argues that because humans are one of the few species that can't synthesize vitamin C, we need relatively large amounts of this nutrient—more than we can possibly get from even the most balanced and healthy of diets. This perspective puts Dr. Pauling at odds with much of the rest of the nutritional and medical establishment in the United States.

Dr. Pauling's reasoning starts with the observation that other species' ability to make huge amounts of ascorbic acid shows that the supply generally available in the diet of humans and animals is insufficient for optimum health. Citing the theories of other researchers, he guesses that about twenty-five million years ago, our ancestors, the evolutionary ancestors of both primates and humans, were able to make vitamin C internally but, through a mutation, lost this ability.

Why did our ancestors lose what would seem like such an advantageous ability? According to the theory Pauling cites, becoming unable to make vitamin C millions of years ago in an unpolluted world filled with plants rich in vitamin C seemed like a good physiological idea at the time. It represented an evolutionary advantage. After all, why waste energy on making ascorbic acid— energy that could be better used for other survival mechanisms—when all the vitamin C an organism such as ours could want was on the nearest berry tree, ripe for the picking?

Dr. Pauling argues that this type of mutation happens all the time among various species. When a mutation presents a severe disadvantage, the mutated forms die out quickly, but when a mutation is advantageous, soon the mutated members of the species predominate. Apparently, in that world of long ago, when vitamin C was plentiful, dropping the burden of making vitamin C meant more chances of survival for our mutant ancestors and their progeny.

From this perspective, when modern humans, descendants of these ancient mutated beings, abandoned a natural diet rich in vitamin C and started dining on foods cooked in ovens and microwaves and desserts dished up with ice cream scoops, we shortchanged our vitamin C requirements.

As part of the proof of this evolutionary argument, Dr. Pauling points to the statements of Dr. Claus W. Jungeblut, an early research pioneer into the uses of vitamin C for strengthening the immune system. Dr. Jungeblut claims that many of our killer diseases may be linked to our lack of vitamin C. How does he know? The guinea pig, which shares our inability to make this nutrient, also shares many of our diseases. Dr. Jungeblut says of the guinea pig, "Of all common laboratory animals, [it] shares with man certain physiological characteristics that include susceptibility not only to scurvy but also to anaphylactic shock, diptheritic intoxication, pulmonary tuberculosis, a poliomyelitislike neurotropic virus infection, and last but not least a form of viral leukemia that is indistinguishable from its human counterpart. None of the vitamin-C-synthesizing laboratory animals (rabbits, mice, rats, hamsters, etc.) answer positively to this call."

This statement implies that all of these diseases might have something to do with the fact that both humans and the guinea pig lack the ability to make vitamin

C. Dr. Pauling doesn't come right out and say it, but he obviously believes that our susceptibility to these diseases might be linked in some way to our refusal to take the amounts of vitamin C that are good for us.

Do these arguments convince many establishment scientists? Not really. Their reaction is, "Don't argue evolution with us, show us some studies that prove we need more of this nutrient." To Dr. Pauling's delight, evidence that supports at least some of his vitamin C advocacy has been accumulating.

Will Vitamin C Make You Live Longer?

One of the more intriguing studies that show that most of us may not be getting the optimum amount of vitamin C was performed by researchers at the School of Public Health at the University of California at Los Angeles. In a large-scale survey that looked at not only the dietary habits of 11,348 people living in all parts of the United States but also measured the vitamin supplements taken by these subjects, the researchers found that, generally speaking, the more vitamin C in people's diet and supplements, the longer they lived.

The folks in this study were followed for ten years. Each time the subjects were contacted, they were asked to recall what they had eaten or swallowed during the past twenty-four hours and also to estimate how often they ate certain foods over a three-month period. Although this is admittedly not a precise way to measure their nutrients, and despite the variables that might have skewed some people's remembrance of the nutrients they were ingesting, the researchers found solid evidence that the vitamin C takers who went way over their RDA for this nutrient had significantly less heart disease and stomach cancer, and they lived longer than those who took lesser amounts.

In this study, vitamin C's wellness effects were particularly striking among men. The fellows taking the most vitamin C had a 42 percent lower mortality rate during the ten years the study went on than the men who took in the least vitamin C. In other words, on a proportional basis, almost twice as many of the vitamin C deprived subjects died as did the vitamin C takers.

Among the women in the study, the big vitamin C takers had a 10 percent lower overall death rate and a 25 percent lower rate of cardiovascular disease than the women who consumed the least amount of vitamin C in their diet or supplements.

In the discussion of their study in the *Journal of Epidemiology*, the UCLA researchers also cited other studies to support their findings. A 1948 survey of elderly residents of San Mateo, California, showed a 50 percent lower death rate among those taking more than 50 milligrams of vitamin C daily. Another study in Almeda, California, showed a 40 percent lower death rate in those taking more than 750 milligrams a day.

While these researchers cautioned that their study did not show that vitamin C specifically prevented disease, they did point out that among the people in their survey, the relationship between consuming very little vitamin C and dying was "stronger and more consistent in this population than the relation of total mortality to serum cholesterol and dietary fat intake, two variables on which strong public health guidelines have been issued over the years."

In other words, their study supported the idea that measuring your vitamin C intake might reveal more about how long you are going to live than measuring your cholesterol or the amount of fat you eat.

Dr. Pauling, of course, would enthusiastically support this kind of conclusion. In his view, how much sucrose—table sugar—you consume and how much vitamin C you take is much more important for your cardiovascular health than worrying about fatty meat. For proof, he cites studies of African tribes that live on fatty milk and meat but suffer very little heart disease. These studies also purportedly show that as these Africans eat more sugar, their rates of heart disease also rise.

The problem with a lot of these population studies are that they reveal associations, but they can't really penetrate into cause and effect linked to nutrients. For instance, just because these people developed more heart disease when they ate more sugar, does that necessarily mean the sugar caused the heart disease? They very well may have been doing some other activity at the same time that was responsible for the increase in this disease.

For example, it could probably be shown that, during this century in the United States, as people have driven their cars more often and at faster speeds, the rate of heart disease and lung cancer has increased. Does that mean that driving a car faster than fifty miles an hour causes heart disease and lung cancer? Not really. It simply means that higher incidences of these diseases have occurred at the same time as this activity, as well as other activities, increase. But those other activities such as driving to the hamburger stand and eating greasy cheeseburgers, or smoking cigarettes while driving, may be responsible for the disease increase.

Vitamin C and Cardiovascular Health

For a long time, Dr. Pauling has believed that ascorbic acid can lower blood pressure. Indeed, several studies show that vitamin C probably does fight hypertension in healthy subjects. And it may be vitamin C's action as an antioxidant vitamin that gives it this capability.

Scientists have theorized that some cases of hypertension are caused in part by damage to the endothelial cells that line the arteries. These special cells help regulate the constriction and relaxation of the arteries. Relaxation lowers blood pressure, while constriction raises it. Free radicals, those reactive molecules liberated by various metabolic processes, may damage these cells so that they remain overly constricted, causing hypertension. This prolonged constriction, aside from causing blood pressure to rise, may also facilitate the deposition of plaque, which can clog the vessels and lead to arteriosclerosis, or hardening of the arteries.

In a study at the Medical College of Georgia in Augusta, researchers discovered that the more vitamin C people had in their blood, the lower their blood pressure. The study, which examined the blood pressure of 168 healthy residents of Augusta who consumed their usual diets, found that those in the group with the most vitamin C in their blood had a mean blood pressure reading of 104/65 millimeters of mercury while those with the lowest amount of this nutrient measured 111/73.

Fifty-six of these people were taking vitamin supplements. Most were taking a multivitamin that contained 60 milligrams of vitamin C (which is the RDA). One person was taking 3 grams a day, and three other people were taking between 200 and 500 milligrams a day.

In their report, these Georgian researchers point out that there are several possible ways vitamin C may lower blood pressure and probably improve your health. In all likelihood, since ascorbic acid is an antioxidant, this helpful nutrient affects the body's production of hormones called prostaglandins. Some of these prostaglandins lower blood pressure by dilating the blood vessels while others have the opposite effect and raise it. These hormones are made from the body's supply of polyunsaturated fatty acids. Apparently, when these acids are oxidized, more of the constricting hormones, which raise blood pressure, may be produced. When vitamin C keeps these fats from being oxidized, it may keep these blood-pressure-raising hormones from flooding the body. In addition, vitamin C may stimulate the production of the dilating hormones that widen the arteries and lower blood pressure.

These Georgian researchers also emphasize that the behavior of the antioxidant vitamins, beta-carotene, vitamin E, and vitamin C, follow a kind of domino pattern. Fall down in your supply of one vitamin, and the available amounts of the others drop. In this case, the presence of ample vitamin C in the blood soaks up free radicals so that together with the vitamin E in the body, vitamin C acts "synergistically . . . in a 'radical crusade.' " Run short of vitamin C, and your vitamin E can't function as well, resulting in increased oxidation of the fats and, possibly, higher blood pressure and heart disease.

Another possible benefit the researchers point to is the power of vitamin C to lower the concentrations of several substances in the blood that may lead to hypertension. These chemicals include sodium, a mineral that, when allowed to float through the blood vessels in excess concentrations, stimulates the release of norepinephrine from various nerve endings and the adrenal glands. Norepinephrine, when it hits the bloodstream, also raises blood pressure.

These researchers also mention one other intriguing fact: The amount of vitamin C found in people's blood also correlates with the amount of fat on their body. Although they say that this relation has yet to be explained, this study and a previous study found that vitamin C blood levels are higher in thinner people. Of course, that doesn't mean that taking this vitamin will make you lose weight, but it does seem to suggest that it couldn't hurt.

Two other investigations, one at Tufts University in Boston and another coordinated with the U.S. Department of Agriculture (USDA) in Maryland, also support the notion that if you have hypertension, you should consider taking vitamin C. The Tufts study of more than 200 Asian-Americans found again that people with the lowest blood pressure tended to have the largest concentrations of vitamin C floating around in their blood. The USDA study showed that twelve people with modest hypertension appeared to benefit from taking a gram of vitamin C a day.

In the USDA research, scientists at Alcorn State University in Mississippi gave the twelve hypertensive men and women 1 gram of vitamin C each day for six weeks. While it is true the vitamin C lowered the systolic blood pressure and not the diastolic (blood pressure is measured with these two numbers: systolic followed by the diastolic; usually the diastolic is considered more important); it was shown that vitamin C reduced the ratio of sodium to potassium in the blood, which could, in the long run, help keep both blood pressure measurements under control.

Vitamin C and Cholesterol

As an extra benefit to the health of your heart and circulatory system, all of the antioxidant vitamins help keep low-density lipoproteins (LDLs), the kind of cholesterol that causes arteriosclerosis, from being oxidized and turned into the evil foam cells that block up arteries. In the role of keeping free radicals from freely gumming up the circulatory system, vitamin C is the champ. In research performed at the University of Texas Southwestern Medical Center in Dallas, it was shown that vitamin C's protective effect against oxidation lasted almost five times as long as did that of vitamin E.

In this Texas study, researchers found that other studies that didn't show a prolonged protective effect for vitamin C simply didn't use enough vitamin C. Although no one really knows how much vitamin C is absorbed by arterial walls and can act to defuse the destructive effects of free radicals, chances are if you consume more than the RDA (60 milligrams a day) of this nutrient, there's a fair amount of it present in these cells. Consequently, it's important to both get your vitamin E and your C. Although the vitamin E in this research provided about five hours of protection, the vitamin C kept inhibiting oxidation to a significant degree for twenty-four hours.

Even though one healthy dose of vitamin C may guard against LDL oxidation for a day or more, it's best to get a sufficient amount of this nutrient every day. Researchers at the University of California at Berkeley have found that oxidation of LDL only begins after the vitamin C in the blood has been used up completely. Although our bodies make special proteins to fight the free radicals that can damage our cells (these special proteins are known to experts as things like catalase and transition-metal-binding proteins), there is a limit to how much of these antioxidant defenders the human body can provide as defense.

That's where the antioxidant vitamins like vitamin C come in. It is much easier to get plenty of vitamin C in food and supplements than it is to flood your body with transition-metal-binding proteins. It probably tastes better too, though the Berkeley researchers are mute on this point.

According to the lab results in Berkeley, vitamin C does not merely provide a modicum of protection against oxidation. As long as this nutrient is present, it seems to provide complete protection, or, as the researchers put it, "Ascorbate [vitamin C] is indeed an outstandingly effective scavenger of aqueous peroxyl radicals." They found that vitamin C was the only antioxidant capable of completely protecting LDLs from being damaged by free radicals, the oxidative bad guys of the body. Once the vitamin C was gone, the other defenders could only offer incomplete protection and some cell structures were at risk of damage.

Vitamin C Concentrates in the Organs

These researchers point out that concentrations of vitamin C in the blood are actually lower than the concentrations in certain of the body's organs that apparently also need antioxidant protection. That probably means that these organs, which include the brain, the liver, the heart, the spleen, the kidneys, the eyes (especially the cornea, lens, and aqueous humor), and the pancreas are not only using vitamin C to help build new tissue but, because these parts of the body have such rapid metabolism, they need vitamin C's protection from free radicals.

In other words, you'll find vitamin C playing an important role every place the body works hardest and uses up lots of oxygen. The processing of oxygen liberates a multiplicity of potentially destructive free radicals. The brain, for instance, while only representing about 2 percent of your body weight, takes up about 18 percent of your body's oxygen consumption and probably generates a wide range of free radicals. The heart, of course, is a metabolic hot spot that is always beating and processing oxygen. Free radicals are let loose in the tissues in your eye every time the eyes are exposed to light.

As a matter of fact, it is circumstances such as these that moved the Dallas researchers to argue that the RDA for vitamin C is significantly too low. The National Research Council advocates 60 milligrams as our daily requirement for vitamin C, but these nutrition scientists believe that an RDA of about 150 milligrams makes more sense for optimal health.

Vitamin C and the Common Cold

The common cold may be common, but it is an annoying disease, nevertheless. Even though it seems like a banal problem, the common cold is actually very complicated. This illness can be caused by a very long list of viruses, and these viruses apparently mutate frequently, changing into slightly different pathogens whose different characteristics confound the search for the elusive cure.

Certainly, many a frustrated cold sufferer who has gone looking for a drug to relieve this affliction has been told that colds usually last about a week, but, with treatment, you can get rid of it in about seven days. Of course, that circular prediction isn't funny when your head throbs, your sinuses ache, your nose runs, and you can't drag your body out of bed. But it does reflect the fact that over-the-counter medications may slightly suppress the symptoms of a cold, but they do nothing to shorten its duration.

Can vitamin C do anything to counter a cold? Dr. Linus Pauling certainly thinks so. Here, once again, there is clinical evidence that tends to support his views.

It was back in 1970 that Dr. Linus Pauling officially opened the whole brouhaha over vitamin C with his book *Vitamin C and the Common Cold.* According to Dr. Jerrold Winter in his book *True Nutrition, True Fitness,* Pauling's argument that taking a few grams of this vitamin each day could keep colds away appealed to vast masses of people because it demonstrated that "a natural substance—said to be totally harmless and able to be purchased without a physician's prescription—would banish the common cold."

At the same time, most medical and nutritional authorities thought that the notion that vitamin C could do anything for a cold or for any other illness was nonsense. Pauling could point to no dependable research showing any effectiveness for vitamin C. Respectable nutrition scientists considered the researchers quoted by Dr. Pauling as disreputable quacks. On top of that, the notion that large dosages of any vitamin could fight off a disease that conventional medicine had been unable to conquer sounded to most scientists like health-nut nonsense, the kind of stuff believed by long-haired people who hang around health food stores. (Remember, this was 1970.)

The objections notwithstanding, after Dr. Pauling's book was published, vitamin C became one of the most popular vitamin supplements, a market position it still holds, second only to multivitamins. The attention raised by the book also led to more thorough investigations of Dr. Pauling's allegations that vitamin C fought off head colds.

Previous to the book's publication, the studies of vitamin C's effect on the common cold had not been rigorous enough to satisfy most scientists, but in 1972, researchers at the University of Toronto began a series of three studies designed to decide once and for all if vitamin C could remedy colds. In the first study, subjects were fed either 1 gram of vitamin C every day or a placebo for a three-month trial. If the subjects began to get a cold during this time, their dosage of vitamin C was bumped up to 4 grams a day for the duration of the illness.

When the experiment started, these Canadian investigators were skeptics. They thought that their study would disprove Pauling's notion that vitamin C had any effect on viral infections of the upper respiratory tract, but they were in for a surprise. When they compared the number of days the placebo group had been sick with the days the people receiving vitamin C were home with a cold, they found the vitamin C group had been incapacitated almost a third less than the control group. This meant that while each group caught just as many colds, the vitamin C group recovered faster and didn't seem to get as sick. This result seemed to show that while vitamin C was hardly a panacea, it did help the body fight off the infection.

In the second Canadian study, the researchers started to get fancy and complicated their procedure. They gave different groups of people different daily doses of vitamin C to see what the various effects would be. This larger study, which involved more than 2,000 people, didn't produce any apparently clear-cut effects of the vitamin. The study contained several groups of people, including two different placebo groups. One of these placebo groups happened to be very healthy during the winter of the study. They hardly got sick at all, and when they did get sick, they recovered quickly. So when this healthy group was compared to the vitamin C groups, it was hard to measure any good the vitamin C had produced. Thus the results were not as encouraging as the first study had been.

The third study got back to basics. In this experiment, everybody either got 500 milligrams a day of the vitamin or a placebo. Among the vitamin takers, those who got a cold immediately received a 1,500-milligram dosage of vitamin C and 1,000 milligrams a day for the duration of the illness. The vitamin takers either took straight vitamin C in tablet form or got it in sustained release capsules. In this test, each group caught about the same number of colds. But a few of the symptoms were not as severe among the group taking the vitamin C. The researchers concluded that vitamin C helped alleviate some cold symptoms but did not prevent colds.

As might be expected, the fact that these tests did not prove that vitamin C was a surefire cure for the common cold left many nonbelievers still not believing in the curative effects of vitamin C. However, there were enough positive results in the studies to keep the true believers truly believing.

As for those who couldn't quite make up their minds, the tests were encouraging. The Canadian study did show that vitamin C was effective much of the time against the common cold. Taking vitamin C could—at least occasionally—keep you from suffering as much or as long from the effects of cold viruses. It may not be a miracle cure, but it works, which is more than you can say for many of the over-the-counter cold symptom remedies advertised by drug companies and pharmacies.

Vitamin C for Athletes

Further research that supports the use of vitamin C to fight infections of the upper respiratory tract has been performed on ultramarathon runners in South Africa. The reason scientists chose this group for a study is these long-distance athletes' high rate of colds and other nose, throat, ear, and bronchial problems that they suffer after running. Apparently, the extreme stress of spending every day training and then spending hours in a race results in quite a few bedridden runners blowing their noses and drinking plenty of fluids.

In this experiment, reported in the *American Journal of Clinical Nutrition,* ninety-two long-distance runners were divided into two groups. Forty-six of the athletes were ordered to take a daily supplement containing 600 milligrams of vitamin C starting three weeks before a ninety kilometer race (the Comrades Marathon, fifty-six miles between Durban and Pietermaritzburg, South Africa). The other runners were given placebo pills containing citric acid without vitamin C.

The results were striking; the incidence of symptoms of upper respiratory tract infection were significantly lower in the runners taking vitamin C. These runners kept taking the vitamin for at least three weeks after the race. (The experimenters also gave vitamins and placebos to an equivalent group of nonrunners. While the members of this group who took vitamin C had the same amount of colds, stuffy noses, and scratchy throats as a placebo group, their symptoms were gone sooner.)

Among the runners, the researchers found that the more runners trained, the more respiratory problems they encountered, but vitamin C seemed to help keep these problems at bay. They believe the reasons for these extra benefits for the runners are probably due to several factors: Exercise uses up vitamin C. Running twelve miles can eliminate about one-fifth of the vitamin C from your blood. Much of this vitamin C is lost in urine and sweat. Also, exercise increases the body's production of free radicals, the oxidative bad guys that attack cell structures. After you exercise, your body may require more antioxidant vitamin C to defuse the destructive threat of these metabolic by-products.

Whatever the explanation, it is clear that vitamin C can help your body fight off colds and keep you breathing clear. If you're an athlete, it's especially important to get some extra helpings of this nutrient.

Long-Term Vitamin C Use

One question these studies don't really answer is the long-term relationship between the colds you get and the vitamin C supplements you take. Each of these studies lasted no longer than three months. Who is to say what happens when you take a gram of vitamin C each day for several years? It is possible that this kind of prolonged regimen might prove even more effective against colds than these short-term treatments. So far, apparently, no one has done long-range tests to see if larger doses of vitamin C taken for several years has a cumulative effect on stopping colds.

If you want to follow Dr. Pauling's advice, you should ingest massive amounts of vitamin C every time you get a cold. According to Dr. Pauling, the appropriate treatment is to take a gram of vitamin C every hour at the first sign of illness. However, he warns that doses this large may cause diarrhea. Still, if it works, a little diarrhea is a fair trade for not getting sick, but as of now there really is no definitive scientific proof that this will work for everybody. After all, not everyone in these studies benefited. It's a bit like chicken soup—it couldn't hurt.

Vitamin C and Cancer

Another controversial area that Dr. Pauling has entered with his vitamin C advocacy is the relationship between vitamin C and cancer. In his books, Dr. Pauling has frequently cited the work of Dr. Ewan Cameron, formerly chief surgeon in Vale of Leven Hospital in Loch Lomondside, Scotland. Beginning in the 1970s, Dr.

Cameron treated many cancer patients with large doses of vitamin C and found, he said, that it helped control pain and, in some instances, kept cancer in check. In his early observations, Dr. Cameron claimed, he had a cancer patient who was taking 12.5 grams of the vitamin every day for twelve years, which successfully suppressed his cancer. Reportedly, every time this patient stopped taking his vitamin C, the cancer returned.

In 1973, Dr. Cameron tried a large-scale study of vitamin C on cancer patients at his hospital. In the trial he gave 100 patients ten grams of vitamin C a day while giving 1,000 other patients a placebo. Within three years, all of the placebo patients had died while 18 of the 100 other patients still survived. At that time, it was reported that, overall, the patients receiving the vitamin C had survived more than four times longer than the control group.

According to Dr. Pauling, these results in Scotland have been replicated in Japan. However, many American scientists have criticized these studies as poorly designed and executed.

Dr. Cameron has his own theories about vitamin C's effectiveness against cancer. He theorizes that vitamin C's activity is related to the fact that cancerous tumors produce an enzyme known as hyaluronidase. This enzyme breaks down the intercellular connective tissue that surrounds the cells of the body. When this intercellular material is weakened sufficiently, the cancerous neoplasm can spread and invade other tissues.

According to this theory, since vitamin C is a coenzyme that promotes the production of collagen, an important component of the intercellular cement holding the body together, this nutrient can help build new connective tissue to replace that broken down during cancer. In addition, vitamin C may act as an enzymatic inhibitor that limits the breakdown action of the hyaluronidase enzyme.

Neither Dr. Cameron nor Dr. Pauling have ever argued that vitamin C is a complete cure for cancer, but both men have argued that it can augment cancer treatment and enable cancer patients to live longer.

The Mayo Clinic Studies Vitamin C

To determine the truth or falsity of these theories about vitamin C and cancer, Charles Moertel at the Mayo Clinic in Rochester, Minnesota, led a large-scale, double-blind study in the late 1970s. In the study, 150 cancer patients received either 10 grams of vitamin C per day or a placebo. To make sure there were no confounding elements that would distort the results of the study, patients in each group were matched by such factors as the type of cancer they had, their age, their sex, and the treatment they had already received.

At the end of this Mayo Clinic experiment, no difference could be found in the condition between the group of patients who had received the vitamin C and the group that had been given the placebos. Thus, the study appeared to show that vitamin C had been of no use whatever in treating these cancer patients.

Dr. Pauling believed otherwise. In his view, the reason the vitamin C had been ineffective was due to the patients' previous treatment with powerful anticancer drugs. He argued that these cytotoxic substances had already damaged the patients' immune systems beyond the point where vitamin C could help them fight off the cancer. He pointed out that few of Dr. Cameron's patients in Scotland (only about 4 percent) had been treated with chemotherapy before taking vitamin C. Finally, he said, the comparison between the placebo group and the vitamin C group was invalid because the placebo group also was consuming more vitamin C than the control groups in Scotland or Japan.

As a result of Dr. Pauling's objections, a follow-up study was conducted at the Mayo Clinic. In this experiment, 100 patients with rectal cancer were given 10 grams of vitamin C per day or a placebo. This time, however, none of the patients in the study had undergone chemotherapy before the start of the clinical trial. Once again, the researchers could find no helpful effect of the vitamin C. In their view, none of the tumors shrank, the cancer progressed just as rapidly in the group receiving vitamin C as it did in the placebo group, and the placebo group lived just as long as the patients who were getting vitamin C.

Dr. Pauling also objected to this study. He believed that these studies were terminated too quickly. In Scotland, he protested, patients took large doses of vitamin C for the rest of their lives—up to fourteen years. In the Mayo study, patients had only been given vitamin C for an average of two and a half months, not enough time to help them. Furthermore, he points out, none of the Mayo patients died while taking the vitamin C. But, instead, their life spans had been measured and compared with the placebo group during the next two years, after they had stopped taking the vitamin.

In Dr. Pauling's view, both the Mayo researchers and the National Cancer Institute suppressed the fact that these patients died after they stopped taking vitamin C. Dr. Pauling believes that a more reliable result could have been had if these cancer victims had been given 10 grams a day of vitamin C for several years.

Is this a case where scientists honestly disagree, or is there a conspiracy to hide the fact that vitamin C is an effective therapeutic tool against cancer? In the book *Vitamin C and Cancer, Medicine or Politics?* Evelleen Richards argues that Dr. Pauling's theories have been the victim of a medical establishment bias against alternative therapies that don't fit in with high-tech, expensive treatments.

For instance, she draws parallels between the inconclusive evidence of vitamin C's effectiveness with the results of trials of the drugs 5-fluorouracil and interferon. Both of these drugs have produced disappointing results when used in seriously ill patients. However, the medical establishment continues to use and test these drugs, which are expensive and often have serious side effects, while brushing aside vitamin C, which is cheap and has virtually no side effects.

In her view, these drugs are a better fit with doctors' need to control patients' therapy. Since they are expensive and must be administered by physicians, they help give doctors added control over patients and their diseases. On the other hand, vitamin C can be bought and taken by anyone. Its holistic milieu goes against the grain of modern medicine.

Ullica Segerstrale in the department of social sciences at the Illinois Institute of Technology, writing in *Science* magazine, offers another perspective: Establishment researchers have more benign reasons for believing that Pauling's arguments for vitamin C are specious. From his perspective, Pauling's arguments are old-fashioned, and smack of the discredited orthomolecular view, which holds that many diseases can be treated well enough if you just throw enough vitamins and herbs at them. In this view, medical researchers are not conspiring against a likely cure, but, instead, are looking to drugs such as interferon and 5-fluorouracil, whose action accommodates more up-to-date theories that focus on chemicals capable of interacting with DNA. These drugs alter the replicative action of the genetic material in the cell nucleus that directs cellular reproduction. Since many medical researchers are convinced that influencing this reproduction will eventually provide the key for curing cancers, they feel more comfortable with chemicals that take this kind of action.

From this perspective, the serious problems with considering vitamin C as a cure for cancer is that it not only does not offer hope as a definitive cure, but it also failed in the two widely publicized trials at the Mayo Clinic. Does that represent a suppression of the facts? According to Dr. Pauling, it does. On the other hand, most people feel that if you discover you have cancer, the standard therapies of drugs and radiation offer better hope for a cure than do massive amounts of vitamins. On his side, Dr. Pauling can produce letters and affidavits from people who claim vitamin C forced their cancer into remission.

Cancer Prevention

As the debate rages over whether or not cancer patients can be helped by vitamin C, evidence is growing that when healthy people eat foods high in this vitamin and take supplements, they may be lowering their risk of ever developing certain cancers.

According to a report by Dr. Gladys Block, a professor of public health and nutrition at the University of California at Berkeley, a review of 180 studies of fruit and vegetable consumption showed that 156 of them found a statistically significant reduced risk of cancer, and the preventive action of vitamin C was especially strong for oral cancer.

As Dr. Block points out, virtually every study that looked at vitamin C consumption found that it reduced the risk of cancer in the mouth. A study performed by the National Cancer Institute in 1988 divided people into four sections according to how much vitamin C they ingested. The people in the top quarter had half the risk for oral cancer of those in the bottom quarter. Other studies show that vitamin C also significantly reduces the risk of cancer in the esophagus and the larynx. These types of cancer most often strike people who smoke and drink alcohol, so the best way to minimize your risk of these kinds of cancer is to give up booze and cigarettes and get your vitamin C. The studies also show that the risk of other cancers such as breast cancer, stomach cancer, and brain cancer are reduced by diets high in vitamin C.

In newspaper stories about breast cancer it is often mentioned that diets high in fat may increase your risk. In the studies on breast cancer cited by Dr. Block, however, it was found that the amount of vitamin C you take in is just as important. As a matter of fact, while saturated fat might increase the risk of this disease, eating fruits and vegetables high in vitamin C reduced the risk by an equal amount.

It was found that children were at greatest risk for brain tumors when their mothers ate little vitamin C. In this research, children born to the 33 percent of women who took in the most vitamin C had only one-third the risk for brain cancer as did other children.

Pollution Fighter

Many studies have looked at vitamin C's ability to help our bodies fight off the effects of pollution. Most of the results of this research—much of it performed on animals—indicates that this nutrient may help offset the harm caused by chemical pollutants we breathe in our air, drink in our water, or eat in our food.

For example, nitrates and nitrites are chemicals commonly found in water and in some cured luncheon meats. They are also found in cigarette smoke and smog. While these chemicals in themselves may not be harmful, when they enter the stomach or lungs, they may be converted into carcinogens called nitrosamines or nitrosourea. However, when vitamin C is present, it interferes with the generation of these chemicals. That is thought to be one important reason vitamin C helps prevent stomach cancer.

Before you have that ham sandwich (the ham may be preserved with nitrates or nitrites), better take your vitamin C, or at least have a slice of tomato, which is high in vitamin C, on the sandwich and down it with a glass of orange juice for some extra helpings of this nutrient.

Smoking and Vitamin C

An additional source of nitrates is cigarette smoke, which is another reason to give up smoking. Along with nitrates, cigarette smoke contains a wide variety of carcinogens, including benzopyrene, a powerful cancer-causing agent used to give cancer to lab animals during experiments.

Because of the stress that smoking puts on the body's immune system, inhaling cigarettes uses up the vitamin C in your body. Some researchers believe that smokers need to ingest more than double the amount of vitamin C that nonsmokers consume in order to keep up the same vitamin C levels in the blood and other tissues.

Before you light up another cigarette to accompany your vitamin supplements, consider one particularly frightening experiment on hamsters who were fed vitamin C and forced to inhale cigarette smoke. The vitamin C given to these animals seemed to speed up the development of some kinds of tumors, even while it appeared to slow the development of others. Admittedly, this kind of test may not be completely analagous to what occurs in humans, but it demonstrates that vitamins are not a panacea for every bad habit.

It's worth repeating again and again: Vitamins are not a cure for poor diet or poor health habits like smoking. Vitamins may improve your health, but quitting smoking, eating a good diet with plenty of fruits and vegetables, getting some exercise, drinking alcohol only in moderation, and dealing reasonably with the stress in your life are important, too. Put these lifestyle habits together with your vitamins, and you will be doing just about all you can to keep yourself in good health. When you are inevitably exposed to someone else's cigarette smoke, or to air pollution, or to some other pollutants in your environment, vitamin C will help your body fight off the effects. Just don't count on vitamin C, or any other nutrient to be a miracle cure.

6

Vitamin D: The Vitamin You Can Make at Home

Some experts take issue with classifying vitamin D as a vitamin. In their view, a nutrient should only be considered a vitamin if it is a substance you need to eat in your diet and that your body can't make. Vitamin D, which comes in two forms, D_2 and D_3 (there is no D_1), is produced in human skin. Any exposure to ultraviolet light or plain old sunshine will cause your skin to make vitamin D. As a matter of fact, some scientists believe that one of the functions of tanning is to shut down the vitamin D production in your skin and prevent overproduction. As melanin, the coloring agent, builds up in the skin cells, less ultraviolet light is permitted through the surface to stimulate vitamin D activity.

Another objection to calling this nutrient a vitamin is the fact that it acts as a hormone in the body, influencing the absorption of calcium from the gastrointestinal tract, and then regulating how calcium is deposited in the bones and other tissues. Most of the other vitamins, in contrast, perform their roles primarily as coenzymes, influencing catalysts for various metabolic processes that may take place more efficiently in their presence.

Despite these scientific objections, vitamin D is still accepted by most experts as a vitamin. It has even received its own official RDA, the official stamp of approval. Among vitamins, however, this nutrient is one of the stranger ones with characteristics and hormonal properties other vitamins don't share.

Rickets: Disease of the City

The fact that vitamin D can be either made in the skin or eaten in the diet confused early researchers who were trying to figure out what made children develop rickets, the young person's deficiency disease caused by a lack of vitamin D. (The adult versions of this disease are called osteoporosis and osteomalacia.) Since vitamin D is necessary for the proper strengthening of bones, this condition is characterized by brittle bones, bones that bend too easily, malformed teeth, and other skeletal abnormalities.

Although rickets had been a recognized disease since ancient times, it was only in the 1800s, when people in northern cities began spending a great deal of time indoors, away from the sun, that rickets began to take on an epidemic significance. Eskimos and others who live on and around the Arctic Circle, where the sun disappears for months at a time, do not have to worry about rickets. The fish that make up a major portion of their diet contains large amounts of vitamin D.

The first European investigations into rickets demonstrated how researchers can miss all the important evidence because of their preconceptions. For instance, it was shown early in the 1800s that dogs raised in darkness developed the disease. At the same time, folk wisdom held that rickets could be cured with cod liver oil (the oil is rich in vitamin D), but establishment doctors chose to ignore or disbelieve both of these keys to the cause and cure of the condition.

Toward the end of the nineteenth century, an English doctor clearly demonstrated that almost everywhere in the world where rickets appeared, it could be linked to a lack of sunlight. It was well known that people who lived on farms never got the disease; only city inhabitants were susceptible. Around the same time, the veterinarians at the London Zoo cured their lion cubs of rickets by feeding them cod liver oil. Despite this convincing evidence of how to cure rickets, the British Royal College of Surgeons was still debating the cause of rickets during World War I, which was about thirty years later.

Even after the war ended, many European scientists believed that rickets was an infectious disease that could be spread by contact. A doctor in Glasgow, Scotland— a city in which rickets was a serious problem—came closer to the truth when he hypothesized that rickets was caused by a lack of fresh air and exercise. He was correct in that fresh air would usually be accompanied by sunshine, the real cure.

It wasn't until relief workers began to work with malnourished children who were suffering the social and economic aftereffects of World War I that the debate over rickets was ended once and for all. In Vienna, Harriet Chick, a British scientist working with an organization called the Accessory Food Factors Committee of the Medical Research Council, established beyond doubt that rickets could be cured with either sunlight, ultraviolet light, or cod liver oil.

It was in the United States during the 1920s that researchers were able to show that fat-soluble vitamin D, while appearing in many foods that also contain fat-soluble vitamin A, had its own distinct identity. It was here in the United States that this vitamin was designated vitamin D.

Vitamin D, the Complex Vitamin

The early researchers who puzzled for years over what caused rickets can be forgiven their confusion when you realize how complicated vitamin D's function is in human nutrition and bone formation. For most people in good health, a very short amount of time in the sun should produce enough vitamin D_3 for proper calcium deposition in the bones.

Unfortunately, many of us who live in northern climes do not get much sunshine since we work indoors in offices, spend much of our leisure time watching TV, bundle up from head to toe for much of the winter, even attend many sports events that are held indoors, and slap on sunscreen whenever we are in the sun. In addition, people with darker skin, whose extra melanin blocks out ultraviolet light, will probably need more sunlight to produce vitamin D than lighter skinned people. This fact leads some scientists to believe that northern humans developed light skin to allow them to synthesize extra vitamin D from smaller amounts of sunshine.

According to the National Research Council, the organization that puts out the RDAs, "Given the many factors that can affect the magnitude of ultraviolet light-dependent synthesis of vitamin D_3, vitamin D should be considered an essential dietary nutrient."

At particular risk of vitamin D deficiency are infants who are breast-fed, don't get out in the sun, and do not receive a multivitamin containing vitamin D; senior citizens whose bodies' production of vitamin D_3 has slowed down; and people who have trouble absorbing vitamin D. If you or someone you know is thought to be suffering from vitamin D deficiency, the victim should consult a doctor and a registered dietitian.

Desist From Vitamin D Megadoses

Because vitamin D can be toxic at high doses, megadosing yourself or your loved ones with this nutrient is an extremely bad idea. If you wish to strengthen your bones, merely taking vitamin D supplements will not achieve this objective.

The relationship between how much vitamin D you ingest and how strong your bones are is not a simple matter. For example, after vitamin D_3 is made in the skin, it doesn't merely stimulate bone formation. Instead, it is first carried to the liver where it is changed into another chemical that is then shuttled off to the kidneys. There it is stored until the parathyroid glands in the neck signal that there is not enough calcium in the blood. The signal from the parathyroid glands consists of a hormone that moves to the kidneys and changes the vitamin D into still another substance that boosts calcium absorption from your food.

Along the way, it is the balance of calcium in your blood, fluctuations in the parathyroid hormone, and regulation by your liver that determines how vitamin D will function in your body. Taking excess vitamin D accomplishes little to change this function and can do harm.

Some of the first evidence of the ill effects of high levels of this vitamin showed up in the 1920s when people began enthusiastically taking big doses. Aside from causing nausea and vomiting and making you lose your appetite, too much of this vitamin can damage your heart and result in calcium deposits in soft tissue. Many victims of vitamin D overdose, especially children, die of kidney failure.

If you are an older adult worried about osteoporosis

or osteomalacia, be warned that a group of older women in Scotland all experienced vitamin D poisoning, or vitamin D intoxication, when they took between 25,000 and 400,000 IU a day. Their symptoms included fatigue and confusion as well as nausea and vomiting. If you are worried about the health of your bones after menopause or at any other time, don't rely on vitamin D supplements, see your doctor for advice.

A real danger with taking large quantities of vitamin D supplements is that many of us take in so much of this vitamin already, that it may be very easy to get too much without realizing it. Milk is supplemented with vitamin D through irradiation with ultraviolet light, which causes the milk to create about 400 IU of this nutrient per quart. That is why the National Research Council, in their statement on the RDAs, warns that "dietary supplements may be detrimental for the normal child or adult who drinks at least two glasses of vitamin D-fortified milk per day."

However, some dark-skinned people who live in northern cities should be aware that in the winter or whenever they spend a great deal of time indoors, they may run into problems with vitamin D deficiency because dark skin is less efficient at producing this vitamin. Deficiencies have arisen occasionally in Scotland and England among African and Pakistani immigrants. In these cases, the answer is usually not to take massive supplements, but merely to include vitamin D fortified milk in the diet or be sure to expose the skin to sunshine every week.

There has also been at least one relatively recent outbreak of rickets in the United States among African American Black Muslim children whose parents followed a strict vegetarian diet. These children spent little time in the sun and their diets included very few foods containing vitamin D. In this case, in Philadelphia, the two dozen children had vitamin D added to their diet and that cured the condition.

Let me remind you once again: If you think you have a serious medical problem such as rickets, osteoporosis, or osteomalacia, see your doctor for a diagnosis. Do not attempt to treat it on your own. Vitamin D supplementation can be dangerous when you take this nutrient in significant amounts.

7

Vitamin A, Beta-Carotene, and the Carotenoids

All animals that have backbones—including humans—have to consume vitamin A in their food or die. Unlike some of the other vitamins, no vertebrate can synthesize vitamin A from scratch. To get a sufficient amount of vitamin A, humans and other species consume what are called vitamin A precursors. These are chemicals in fruits and vegetables that the body readily converts to vitamin A as needed.

The vitamin A precursors are known as carotenoids, pigmented substances that make carrots yellow, pink grapefruit pink, and give many other vegetarian foods such as apricots, mangoes, and papayas their characteristic colors. Of the 500 known carotenoids, about 50 can be made into vitamin A in the body. Of these vitamin A precursors, the one that seems to be the most important for the human body is beta-carotene. In the lingo of nutrition scientists, beta-carotene seems to have the greatest "biological activity." It is the most readily converted to vitamin A but, while it is waiting for possible conversion, it doesn't just stand there, it does something—and the something that it does is very beneficial for your body. The biological activity of the other carotenoids are less well understood but it is believed that they are not used as efficiently as beta-carotene.

Seeing the Benefit of Vitamin A

One of vitamin A's most important tasks in the body is to help with night vision. When your eyes are trying to see objects in dim light, they make use of a chemical called vitamin A aldehyde, a derivative of vitamin A. When your diet starts to seriously run low on vitamin A, you may notice that darkness seems darker and objects that used to be easy to see disappear into murkiness.

Vitamin A also plays a crucial role in the formation of epithelial tissue, the tissue that surrounds the cavities of the body. Epithelial tissue makes up your skin, lines the intestines, the stomach, the throat, and the urogenital tract, and it forms an important part of your eyes. When you are seriously deficient in vitamin A, your body suffers dire consequences: Your bones, your reproductive organs, your skin, and your respiratory tract all begin to malfunction.

In addition, you need sufficient vitamin A to maintain your immune system, the protective cells in your body that fight off foreign microbial invaders that can make you sick. One reason malnourished inhabitants of Third World countries are more frequently threatened by infectious diseases than are citizens of the better-fed United States is that they lack vitamin A in their diet. For example, a study in Africa showed that when malnourished children were fed vitamin A supplements, the measles fatality rate dropped dramatically. Similarly, a recent study of children in southern India showed that a small, weekly dose of vitamin A cut the overall child mortality rate by more than 50 percent.

We Don't Need Much Vitamin A

Fortunately, few Americans suffer from vitamin A deficiency. While it is estimated that every year vitamin A deficiency causes 500,000 corneal lesions in children throughout the world (these lesions are hardening of parts of the eye, a condition that can cause blindness), it is extremely rare to find an American adult threatened by vitamin A deficiency. If you have any question about your vitamin A intake, a simple multiple vitamin can fulfill your needs.

There is little reason to take large doses of this nutrient. Many medical people believe that megadoses of vitamin A can be toxic, although other vitamin experts such as Linus Pauling dispute its toxicity. According to the National Research Council, the organization that oversees the RDAs, in order to overdose on vitamin A, you would usually have to take high doses over an extended period of time. Adults have to take 50,000 IU or more daily, while infants and young children would have to ingest more than 20,000 IU a day. That is approximately ten times the RDA.

Usually, the only people who get into trouble by taking too much vitamin A are those who take vitamin supplements and also eat a diet high in liver or fish oil, both of which are very high in vitamin A. The symptoms of getting too much vitamin A include headache, vomiting and nausea, dry mouth and dryness of mucous membranes, liver damage, bone abnormalities, diplopia, and alopecia.

Beta-Carotene: Safer for You Than Vitamin A

Beta-carotene, the vitamin precursor that your body can convert into vitamin A, has been the subject of some of the most exciting research examining vitamins and human health. Even though beta-carotene has to be converted into vitamin A before the body can use it to fulfill your vitamin A requirement, in many ways, beta-carotene appears to be a superior nutrient to vitamin A.

One big advantage of beta-carotene is its low toxicity. Vitamin A can cause discomfort and possible organ damage when taken in large amounts, but beta-carotene seems to be virtually risk-free, even when ingested in extremely large doses. Usually, the only reported side effect caused by large, extended dosages of beta-carotene is a yellowish tinge to the skin. What seems to happen is that beta-carotene, the pigment that makes carrots yellow, can make your skin turn yellow or orange when you megadose yourself for a few weeks. This effect is especially noticeable in the palms of your hands and the soles of your feet.

This orangish skin coloring is considered harmless, although you might find it embarrassing to have hands that look like a carrot. However, there is one downside to megadosing beta-carotene. If you are also a heavy drinker, the beta-carotene supplements may put a strain on your liver. A study at the Veterans Affairs Medical Center in New York found that heavy drinking combined with daily 30-milligram doses of beta-carotene inflamed the livers of baboons. The baboons drank the equivalent of about a pint of liquor a day. The 30 milligrams of beta-carotene represents the amount of beta-carotene in about half a pound of carrots.

According to the researchers, the lesson we should take from this study is to cut down on the alcohol, not on the beta-carotene. They believe that in humans a combination of prolonged heavy drinking and beta-carotene supplementation could cause liver abnormalities.

Beta-Carotene Quenches Free Radicals

If beta-carotene were only a vitamin A precursor, it might not be too important in human nutrition. However, research has shown that being turned into vitamin A is only one of its roles in the body. It has many other important duties to perform.

Even if your body has sufficient vitamin A and doesn't convert the beta-carotene you've taken into retinol (retinol is the chemical name for vitamin A), apparently the beta-carotene that travels through your body can help stave off some forms of cancer and heart disease.

Plants manufacture beta-carotene and other carotenoids to protect themselves from oxidation. Green plants containing chlorophyll use the energy in sunlight to convert water and oxygen into useful fuel for growing and survival. This process, known as photosynthesis, not only produces food, it liberates singlet oxygen, a kind of cellular pollution, which, if allowed to react with the cells in leaves, roots, and stems, would quickly kill the plant.

One of the first medical uses in humans for beta-carotene evolved from researchers' knowledge of its function as an antioxidant in plants. In the late 1960s and early 1970s, patients with a genetic disease called erythropoietic protoporphyria, whose skin was supersensitive to light, were given beta-carotene to see if the chemical could protect them. In most cases it worked. This was one of the first indications that beta-carotene could prevent or treat disease in humans.

Double Bonds That Preserve Health

According to Norman I. Krinsky, Ph.D., professor of biochemistry and pharmacology at Tufts University, beta-carotene quenches singlet oxygen by dissipating its destructive energy throughout the carotenoid molecule. Beta-carotene is able to do this because it possesses a chemical bond arrangement known as conjugated double bonds. When it meets singlet oxygen, the oxygen's energy reverberates over beta-carotene's bonding arrangement and is released in the form of heat. As this very small amount of heat is released, the singlet oxygen is converted to a less destructive form of oxygen that is less likely to form free radicals.

Singlet oxygen, in and of itself, is not a free radical. It forms free radicals when it transfers energy to another molecule in the cell's protoplasm. Free radicals are highly reactive, electrically charged molecules that contain unpaired electrons. When electrons are unpaired, they tend to either be discharged into other molecules or they pull out neighboring electrons from other substances. This action destabilizes the structures or membranes of the cell.

The reaction of a free radical with cellular structures can start a chain reaction of destruction as more free radicals are generated and important parts of the cell are chemically torn to pieces.

Attack on the Lipids

Many of the lipids—special types of fats—that circulate through the body are in liquid form. These lipids have what are called unsaturated chemical bonds, open-ended chemical bonds that are particularly vulnerable to attack by free radicals. If the bonds were saturated, the fats could not circulate because they would solidify.

When the lipids in cell membranes come under attack by free radicals, the chain reaction can be severe enough to kill the cell. Experimentally, scientists have established that beta-carotene, as well as another carotenoid known as canthaxanthin, can guard membranes against this kind of damage. (Canthaxanthin is similar to beta-carotene, but it cannot be converted into vitamin A.)

A startling experiment that demonstrates the power of beta-carotene's protective powers involved injecting guinea pigs with carbon tetrachloride. This rather obnoxious chemical causes what is called lipid peroxidation, a free radical reaction that tears up lipids. Guinea pigs who had been given beta-carotene suffered much less damage than did guinea pigs without this carotenoid.

Since we live in a seriously polluted environment and are exposed to chemicals similar to carbon tetrachloride (though not in such drastic doses as these laboratory animals were given) it could be argued from studies like this that we need beta-carotene to ward off the oxidative effects of industrial chemicals. Some researchers believe that a combination of beta-carotene, vitamin E, and vitamin C are a necessity to survive the free radicals we all meet in everyday life.

Beta-Carotene Versus Arteriosclerosis

A study at the Harvard Medical School indicates that daily doses of beta-carotene may delay or prevent hardening of the arteries, the condition known as arteriosclerosis. The study reported in *Science News* involved giving 50-milligram doses of beta-carotene every other day to men who suffered from angina, the chest pain associated with heart disease.

Previous to this study, animal experiments had shown that antioxidant drugs, which disarm the destructive power of free radicals, had the potential for retarding the development of arteriosclerosis. For example, a study in 1988 demonstrated that rabbits born with a genetic defect making them susceptible to arteriosclerosis would have their risk of hardening of the arteries cut in half when given antioxidant drugs. But no one knew whether or not antioxidant vitamins would cut that risk in animals or in humans.

The Harvard study was a classic double-blind study. Half of the 333 men in the study were given beta-carotene pills, and the other half were given placebos, pills that contained inactive ingredients. This type of experiment is called a double-blind study because neither the subjects in the study nor the people giving them their pills know which pills are real and which are fake. The purpose of a double-blind study is to reliably establish the effectiveness of the substance being tested. If the group receiving placebos are benefited as much as the group receiving the vitamin or drug being studied, then the researchers conclude the test showed the substance is without usefulness.

In the research at Harvard, which went on for six years, the group of heart patients who received the 50-milligram beta-carotene pills fell victim to only half as many strokes, heart attacks, and other cardiovascular difficulties as did the men who received placebos.

According to William A. Pryor, a vitamin researcher at Louisiana State University and a longtime advocate of the usefulness of using vitamins to prevent chronic diseases, this Harvard study represents a "gold standard proof that physicians have been waiting for." Pryor believes that this research is the first that firmly establishes the effectiveness of using antioxidants to ward off arteriosclerosis.

8

Vitamin E: The Mountain-Climbing Vitamin

Skeptics have often referred to vitamin E as the vitamin in search of a disease. This skepticism is largely based on two facts: A clear-cut vitamin E deficiency is hard or impossible to induce in normal adults, and, for a long time, no one could quite figure out exactly what vitamin E was supposed to do in the human body. Years ago, some researchers claimed vitamin E had miraculous powers in preventing angina, but this power—without the presence of other vitamins—could not be firmly proven in follow-up tests. That just gave the skeptics more ammunition for their diatribe against this vitamin.

While the history of vitamins is replete with dread deficiency diseases such as beriberi, rickets, scurvy, and pellagra that plagued populations around the world, there has never been an equally frightening epidemic of vitamin E deficiency. You can scrape by on very little of this nutrient. You may not be in optimum health if you don't get much vitamin E, but you won't appear to be sick. If you're a typical American, you will be as vitamin E sufficient as your neighbor, who also probably does not get much of this vitamin.

To nutrition researchers, trying to induce vitamin E deficiency in test subjects is the scientific equivalent to beating your head against the wall. In one study, performed in the 1950s, a researcher tried unsuccessfully for six years, (that's right, six years) to produce vitamin E deficiency in nineteen volunteers.

To give you an idea of how volunteers for medical studies have suffered in the name of nutrition science, consider that during the first two years of this study the volunteers ate, as their only source of fat, lard that had had the vitamin E removed. When two years of lard didn't put them into vitamin E deficiency (their blood levels still showed some vitamin E and they weren't suffering from any symptoms that could be pinned on lack of vitamin E), the lard was taken out of their diet and they were fed corn oil without vitamin E. Four years on the corn oil diet didn't do it, either. Of course, they were eating other foods during this entire time, but nothing with any appreciable vitamin E in it. After six years, the researchers gave up and let the subjects go back to eating the diet of their choice.

In light of this frustrating experiment, who can we say ever develops a vitamin E deficiency? According to the National Research Council, the folks who cook up the RDAs, there are two significant cases when E deficiency causes overt, serious problems: Premature infants of very low birth weight develop medical difficulties due to lack of this nutrient (they develop a particular type of anemia among other things), and children and adults who don't absorb fat normally. Cystic fibrosis is linked, at least in part, to an inability to absorb vitamin E.

Eat Your Fat, but Make It the Right Kind

Although many dietitians, nutritionists, and researchers have been trying to persuade Americans to eat less fat, the fatty diet we consume has one advantage: It often contains vitamin E. The polyunsaturated fats, such as corn oil, contain this nutrient. That means that some people who cut back on fat may also be cutting back on vitamin E.

The fact that vitamin E is in vegetable oils comes in handy because when your body absorbs fat from your food, destructive, oxidative free radicals are set loose, and the body needs vitamin E to deal with these molecular bad guys.

In order to get vitamin E from your diet, you must not eat entirely fat-free meals and snacks. That doesn't mean you should pig out on all the fatty foods you can stomach, but it does mean that if you neglect the oil in your diet, you'll also be cutting back on vitamin E. Don't count on fatty meats for this nutrient. The National Research Council points out that meats, fish, animal fats, and most fruits and vegetables have little vitamin E. Leafy green vegetables, however, are a good source of the nutrient.

Originally, when vitamin E research was in its dark ages, scientists found that rats fed rancid fats were unable to have baby rats. Rancid fats are fats that have been oxidized. This oxidation process uses up all the vitamin E in the fat when the vitamin is converted to other substances in the oily struggle to stop the oxidation.

In these early experiments, the scientists found that when these fat-eating rats were fed lettuce along with their diet of rancid fat, it was like giving them a fertility drug. They regained the power to reproduce. The unknown fertility factor in the lettuce that restored rat reproductive ability was thereupon named factor X.

Factor X, it was soon shown, wasn't just in lettuce. Wheat germ oil was also found to contain this factor. As researchers made progress in isolating this factor, they took its X away from it and started calling it vitamin E. It was also called tocopherol, from the Greek words meaning *carry* and *childbirth,* since the vitamin had been shown to be necessary in rat fertility.

Eventually, it was discovered that there were several versions of the tocopherols primarily contained in vegetable oils, wheat germ, nuts, seeds, and leafy green vegetables. These were named alpha-, beta-, gamma-, and delta-tocopherol. Another group of compounds, the tocotrienols, were also found. However, of all these forms of vitamin E, alpha-tocopherol, which is most prevalent in food, is also the most active form of vitamin E and is most useful in human nutrition.

Because vitamin E was found to be helpful to rodents trying to have babies, early vitamin enthusiasts promoted this vitamin as a fertility aid. Despite these claims, so far there isn't any evidence to show that this nutrient will help you have children if you are unable to do so now.

Vitamin E and Cancer

What are the other reasons the alleged health benefits of vitamin E turn so many nutrition researchers into skeptics? Inflated claims for this nutrient by vitamin marketers have turned many of these folks into scientists with an attitude—an anti–vitamin E attitude. Some vitamin sellers have claimed this substance (actually a group of closely related substances known as tocopherols) can cure impotence, improve muscular dystrophy, alleviate rheumatic fever, and clear up varicose veins. No research has upheld these claims. Unfortunately, for a long time, the snake oil advertising for this vitamin seems to have made scientists ignore this antioxidant. As one doctor snidely put it, the uses of vitamin E are limited only by the imagination.

Lately, researchers are coming up with solid proof of the vitamin's usefulness. What they often seem to find is that vitamin E is most effective in conjunction with other antioxidants such as vitamin C and beta-carotene in fighting off free radical destruction in the body. One reason early researchers may have had a hard time discovering how a lack of vitamin E affects health was that they didn't look at how vitamin E functions as a partner with the other antioxidant vitamins.

Studies indicate that to do its job of antioxidant protection, vitamin E itself needs to be protected by the presence of other antioxidants. What that means is that when free radicals are let loose in the blood or in other tissues, defusing their destructive power can quickly use up the available vitamin E. When substances like vitamin C and beta-carotene are also present, vitamin E's antioxidant abilities may be prolonged. Together, these antioxidants may act synergistically, each helping the other to protect the body in powerful ways that they are unable to accomplish by themselves.

The apparent synergistic action of the antioxidants may make them into a powerful force against cancer. To verify this effect, a study measured the blood levels of vitamin E, beta-carotene, and vitamin C in healthy people living in Maryland, and then kept tabs on these people for two years to see who would develop lung cancer. The researchers found that those with the lowest amounts of these nutrients in their blood had twice the risk of developing lung cancer as people with the highest levels.

Similar findings resulted from a study of cervical cancer. Researchers found that when diets were high in vitamin E, vitamin C, and beta-carotene, people had half the risk of cervical cancer as did others who ate little of these substances.

Still other studies demonstrate the same effect. A survey looking at oral cancer in African-Americans found that those with diets high in vitamin E had half the risk of cancer as others. A wide survey in Finland found that Finns who ate foods rich in vitamin E had one-fourth to one-fifth the risk of stomach, urinary, and pancreatic cancers as those who didn't eat those kinds of foods.

Vitamin E Fights Oxidative Stress

Although vitamin E functions synergistically with other antioxidants, in many tissues of the body it is the vitamin E that is the principal agent in cutting short the potent destruction of free radicals. Free radicals, harmful molecular products of normal metabolism that attack cell structures, are generated during virtually every cellular activity.

Interestingly enough, both smoking and aerobic exercise are forms of oxidative stress that increase your exposure to free radicals. Smoking introduces free radicals into your body in the smoke you inhale. Aerobic exercise is healthier for you than smoking since it builds up muscles and cardiovascular endurance, but the increase in metabolic processes and muscle activity during exercise also causes an increase in free radicals. Both of these activities can increase your need for vitamin E and the other antioxidants.

To measure how athletes are affected by vitamin E and oxidative stress, researchers in Europe measured the amount of pentane in the breath of mountain climbers while they were scaling the peaks. Pentane is a gas that is made when fats are oxidized. Measured in the breath, pentane increases when more oxidation is taking place in the body.

The researchers found that when they gave mountain climbers 1,000 IU of vitamin E a day for a month, they did not experience the kind of increases in pentane in their breath while climbing that occurred without taking the vitamin. Researchers believe this result shows that the vitamin E was probably beneficial in cutting down on the oxidative stress taking place in their bodies. This is the same kind of stress that jogging, biking, aerobic dance, or long walks can generate.

Vitamin E and Heart Disease

When it comes to vitamin E's relationship to heart disease, most conservative researchers have, at least in the past, downplayed its effectiveness. That's because studies seemed to show that vitamin E could not relieve the discomfort of patients with angina, the chest pain that many people with heart disease get when they exert themselves.

More recent research demonstrates that this nutrient is vital for the health of your heart, whether or not you suffer from heart disease. Once again, the latest studies seem to show that frequently it is the combined levels of more than one of the antioxidant vitamins, vitamins E and C and beta-carotene, that may be important for your health.

When scientists at the University of Edinburgh in Scotland studied the blood of about 500 men, 100 of whom had angina, they found that the men with chest pain tended to have lower blood levels of these nutrients, particularly of vitamin E. These researchers believe that men who eat foods containing beta-carotene and vitamin C (fruits and vegetables) as well as foods containing vitamin E such as whole grains, nuts and seeds, and vegetable oils, take in more nutrients that protect their hearts. On the other hand, they state, the fact that middle-aged Scots eat so little produce may be a factor in giving Scotland a very high rate of heart disease.

Keeping Platelets Apart

One way vitamin E may help heart disease patients is through its interaction with cells in the bloodstream called platelets. Platelets are important for healing cuts and wounds. Without them, we might bleed to death. Every time you suffer a tear or break in your skin and start to bleed, platelets stick to the injured flaps of skin, stick to each other, and clump together to plug the injury.

As the platelets begin to stick together, they release prostaglandins, chemical signals in the plasma that increase their stickiness even more, until the broken blood vessels are closed off. Technically speaking, this forms a thrombosis, which staunches the blood flow.

When the platelets are functioning normally, they are a lifesaver, but the process can malfunction in harmful ways. The platelets can get sticky and clump together (aggregate) in the bloodstream at inappropriate times, when there is no cut to be healed. This can lead to the formation of blood clots that can potentially stick in the heart, lungs, or brain, causing a heart attack or stroke. Sometimes these clots can block arteries in the arms or legs and initiate or accelerate the collection of athero-sclerotic plaque, the fatty deposits that coat arteries and impede circulation.

Research demonstrates that vitamin E can help platelets function normally, decreasing the likelihood of trouble-some clots. In the lab, vitamin E has been shown to slow down platelets' release of prostaglandins, the chemical group that makes these cells stickier.

Some scientists think that vitamin E influences platelet function by directing its antioxidant power against an acid that oxidizes when the platelets begin to clump together.

If allowed to oxidize, this substance, called arachidonic acid, may form another prostaglandin that makes platelets stickier.

Platelets carry around their own supply of vitamin E, but as you get older, the amount of vitamin E contained in your platelets drops, which may be one reason for increased heart disease in the aged. There is evidence, however, that taking vitamin E supplements can at least partially offset this decline.

In another experiment, it's been shown that when people took 400 IU a day of vitamin E, their platelets had less of a tendency to stick to collagen, a substance inside the lining of the blood vessels. This is important, because collagen is exposed when blood vessels are injured. With less of a tendency to stick to an injury in a blood vessel, the chances of the platelets starting a blood clot are decreased.

Vitamin E and Aspirin

Today, many heart patients are taking aspirin every day. Studies have demonstrated that aspirin lowers the chance of harmful blood clots by decreasing the gathering of platelets, although the mechanism for this action has not been satisfactorily explained. However, it has been shown that aspirin has no effect on platelet adhesion or stickiness. Since vitamin E does decrease stickiness, its action may be able to complement and increase the protective action of aspirin for these people.

As a further benefit, some researchers have found that vitamin E also helps control blood clotting in insulin-dependent diabetics who may be at increased danger from platelet activity. In a double-blind test where some diabetics received either placebos or vitamin E, investigators discovered that vitamin E cut back on platelet grouping and also inhibited the release of prostaglandins. A survey of diabetics showed that the ones with the stickiest platelets had the lowest levels of vitamin E in their blood.

When Blood Flows Back In

Cutting off the blood supply to a part of the body has serious repercussions. When a limb loses circulation, gangrene can set in as tissue dies. That can necessitate amputation. If the blood supply is cut off to a part of the brain, a stroke occurs. When a section of the heart is cut off from its blood supply, either angina (chest pain) or a heart attack may result. This deficiency in blood supply because of a blockage or constriction of a blood vessel is called ischemia.

Surgical procedures that resupply blood to deprived areas are called reperfusion. After some heart attacks, reperfusion is accomplished by using drugs to break apart blood clots that restrict blood flow to the heart.

Reperfusion procedures restore circulation but often cause a degree of further tissue damage by temporarily increasing the concentration of free radicals in the affected part of the body. When the free flow of oxygenated blood suddenly floods the blood vessels, the overwhelming number of free radicals that are set loose is too much for cellular defense mechanisms. Consequently, severe damage may result.

According to Donald Mickle, M.D., deputy biochemist-in-chief at the Toronto Hospital, "Vitamin E is our major, and possibly only, membrane-soluble antioxidant able to prevent this damage." Apparently, high levels of vitamin E may be able to defuse the oxidative destructive force of these molecular marauders. So far, much of the work in this area has explored the use of vitamin E to prevent heart damage in animals. Water-soluble forms of vitamin E are being perfected for injection into heart attack patients.

Meanwhile, other researchers have tried giving high doses of vitamin E to heart bypass patients. During bypass operations, hearts are put on ice and temporarily relieved of their job of pumping blood while surgeons reroute blood vessels around arterial blockages. After the procedure, hearts may be injured when they are restarted and blood flow resumes through them.

During one study, ten bypass patients received 2,000 IU of vitamin E about twelve hours before their operations. During the surgery, they showed no increase in their blood levels of hydrogen peroxide, a marker that indicates oxidative stress in the body. Other patients, who didn't receive the vitamin, showed much higher levels of hydrogen peroxide.

Getting the extra vitamin E also helped the patients retain vitamin E in their blood after the operations. Patients without the vitamin supplements had sharp drops in vitamin E blood levels a day after bypass.

Vitamin E Eases Some Types of Pain

In some people, problems with their blood vessels, such as the plaque buildup in atherosclerosis, may not completely cut off blood supply to certain areas of the body, but it can reduce it enough to cause pain and numbness in limbs as well as muscle cramping and fatigue. For these people, too, vitamin E may bring relief, although it is not an infallible cure.

In a study of these types of problems, two-thirds of the subjects who had poor circulation in their legs (a condition called intermittent claudication) had some of their pain and cramping relieved with the use of vitamin E. In another experiment, patients with poor circulation in their lower legs took vitamin E and were encouraged to give up smoking and start exercising. After two years, the blood flow to their lower legs had increased by an average of 34 percent, while patients who had been taking drugs but no vitamin E had no improvement in their circulation. The patients taking vitamin E could also walk farther, on average, than the people not taking the vitamin.

Of course, these test results do not mean that you should ever treat a serious medical problem such as leg pain or muscle problems by yourself. Talk to your doctor about the most appropriate treatment. These studies show that vitamin E can help patients, but serious problems demand serious medical care.

Vitamin E and Your Immune System

The human immune system consists of a complicated amalgamation of cells that communicate with each other, help each other battle infectious agents, and are capable of reproducing rapidly in response to the threat of disease. It has been relatively easy for researchers to show that vitamin E boosts the immune systems of animals. Many studies have shown that on the farm and in the lab, animals fed vitamin E supplements do not get sick as easily or as often as animals that do not take this nutrient.

For example, in a study of mice with an often fatal type of pneumonia, the rodents who received substantial doses of vitamin E survived more often than did mice who received less of the vitamin. In research comparing young mice to old, the supplemented senior mice who would normally have had weaker immune systems than young mice demonstrated better immune responses on all tests compared to young mice who didn't take vitamins.

In people, it has been a little harder to pin down whether or not vitamin E enhances immunity and, if it does, exactly how it works. But in looking at the human immune response, scientists recognize that the makeup of the cells involved would seem to indicate that vitamin E must be important.

For one thing, immune cells often communicate with each other through releases of chemicals (lipids and proteins) that have to cross membranes, those thin little envelopes that surround all cells. Because immune activity involves so many membranes, the integrity of membranes—their freedom from damage—is essential to the proper functioning of immunity.

Since membranes are often made up of lipids, the chief enemy of these coverings are free radicals that act to oxidize and break down membranes' components. As a result, antioxidants like vitamin E are important for keeping these substances from being destroyed by reactive molecules. When vitamin E is low, membranes are more vulnerable to destruction. Researchers believe that vitamin E protects these lipids and the polyunsaturated fatty acids that are abundant in the immune system cells.

Another important function for vitamin E seems to be in aiding the reproduction of immune cells. The cells that are the main workers of the immune system multiply rapidly when faced with an invasion of disease-causing pathogens. This process, called mitogenesis, gives them a vast defensive power.

In a study of women who had trouble absorbing vitamin E from their diet and who had very low levels of vitamin E in their blood, researchers found that there were also extremely low levels of substances needed to help immune cells reproduce. To test how this deficiency affects the immune system, the scientists performed skin tests. In the tests, an injection just under the skin demonstrates sensitivity to foreign substances. The women who had low levels of vitamin E had skin that showed virtually no immune response at all.

After these women were given vitamin E supplements for a week, their immune systems seemed to wake up from their stupor. Skin tests showed positive responses (where before there had been none) and blood tests showed increased functioning of immunity-related activity. According to researchers, this response in humans corresponds with the observation that when you give vitamin E to any animal over and above the recommended amounts, immune systems are revved up and more prepared to cope with and defeat disease.

Old Immune Systems

As you age, your immune system doesn't necessarily get better, it often gets slower and less responsive to foreign invaders. A frequent sign of impaired immunity is in the formation of lipid peroxide. This reflects oxidation of the fatty acids in cellular membranes and corresponds with reduced effective immune response. This slowdown in immunity has been blamed for the increased vulnerability of the aged to disease and infirmity. Consequently, when you get old, you get sick more often, and each time you get sick you also get sicker. Resistance to the formation of tumors and cancer also may be impaired when you get older. Your body slowly may lose the ability to fight off the problems it would have shrugged off easily when you were younger.

To investigate the idea that the state of your aging immune system may be dangerous to your health, researchers in the Southwest did a seven-year study on 300 New Mexican senior citizens who were in apparent good health. At the beginning of the study, all the subjects took a skin test designed to show the sensitivity of their immune systems. By the end of the study, the folks who had initially displayed the least response to the skin test were twice as likely to have died as the other people.

When researchers in France studied the vitamin E levels in the blood of older French citizens, they found that senior citizens with higher amounts of circulating vitamin E became ill fewer times over a period of two to three years than did people with less vitamin E.

In another study, this one a double-blind test where half the test subjects were given vitamin E supplements while the other half were given capsules that only looked like vitamin E, people over the age of sixty who took 800 IU a day for a month showed much higher immune reactions. In this particular study, vitamin C and beta-carotene did not seem to increase sensitivity on a skin test or produce other signs of increased immune response as did vitamin E.

Vitamin E and Cataracts

Cataracts, an eye problem common to aging, occur when a section of the lens hardens and becomes opaque. Usually cataracts can be removed surgically and, with the aid of thick glasses, most cataract victims still have adequate vision after this operation.

Although cataract operations have been performed for more than 100 years, until relatively recently, little has been known about how the cataract process begins. Under normal circumstances, the eye's lens is flexible and transparent. What causes it to harden and become useless?

Once again, the villains that cause the cellular damage to the body have been found to be free radicals. Many studies indicate that the combination of oxidative stress that takes place in the eye combined with the reduction of available antioxidants as you get older lays the groundwork for the construction of cataracts.

The eye, it turns out, faces a constant danger from free radicals every moment you are awake. Because every time light strikes your eyes the energy from the light liberates these reactive molecules that can attack your lens.

While studies of animals have strongly shown vitamin E to have a protective effect against cataracts, slowing down their progress and damage, the evidence in human studies indicates that this nutrient probably needs some help to protect your eyes. It cannot do the job alone. When researchers measured how well vitamin E could protect human eyes from cataracts, they found that it seemed to help somewhat, but when they looked at the combined effect of vitamin E along with the antioxidants vitamin C and beta-carotene, they found a significant decrease in the risk of cataracts.

Of course, none of this evidence shows that vitamin E or any of the other antioxidant vitamins can be used to treat cataracts. Once these lesions form in the eye, medical intervention is almost always necessary. Certainly, if you think you are having any kind of serious problems with your eyes, you should consult a doctor. However, if you want to lower your risk of someday developing cataracts, taking these vitamins may help.

Anemia and Vitamin E

Another area that shows promise for vitamin E use is to treat people suffering certain types of anemic conditions. Anemia is a lack of red blood cells. When these cells are destroyed at a high rate in your body, the condition is called hemolytic anemia. Some scientists believe that oxidation of the membranes of these cells by free radicals may be a factor that worsens this condition.

Therefore, if vitamin E can help keep these membranes intact by resisting oxidative destruction, it will alleviate this problem.

Investigations of this disease have shown that people who suffer chronic hemolytic anemia have low levels of alpha-tocopherol in their blood. When doctors gave these patients 800 IU of vitamin E a day for a year, their red blood cells lasted longer and some symptoms of their anemia decreased. Children suffering this disease also seemed to improve when given the same amount of vitamin E.

Sickle cell anemia is another condition that shows promise of being at least partially alleviated with vitamin E. In this disease, some red blood cells assume an odd sickle form. Instead of taking on the usual sort of round, concave, lifeboat shape that red blood cells are supposed to have, many of the cells elongate and twist. The more cells that assume this deformed shape, the more serious the disease.

Sickle cell anemia is also peculiar in that some red blood cells go from being misshapen to assuming a normal shape after they pick up a supply of oxygen from the lungs. Other twisted cells, however, remain deformed no matter what the circumstances. The more cells that are irreversibly misshapen, the more red blood cell destruction takes place in the body and the worse the anemia becomes.

A study in which sickle cell anemia patients were given 450 IU of vitamin E a day showed that the number of permanently sickled cells decreased from 25 percent of red blood cells to around 10 percent. Another study showed similarly positive results when patients were fed 400 IU a day.

Besides preserving more normal red blood cells, vitamin E benefited the immune systems of those with sickle cell anemia. In another study, blood drawn from sickle cell sufferers showed low levels of vitamin E as well as an increased tendency to form oxygen free radicals. Supplementation with vitamin E seemed to improve their immune systems and boosted their resistance to these molecular marauders.

Of course, if you think you are suffering from any form of anemia, you should consult your doctor to find the cause and be treated. If you are currently being treated for anemia, you should talk to your physician about the possible benefits of taking vitamin E.

High Doses of Vitamin E

In the past, the conventional wisdom held that water-soluble vitamins were safer to take in large doses over a long period of time than fat-soluble vitamins. The rationale for this belief was based on the fact that fat-soluble vitamins can usually be stored for quite a while in the body's fat. Therefore, the theory went, the fat-soluble vitamins A, D, E, and K had a better chance of building up in large quantities and causing toxicity, poisoning the body as the physiological systems used for storing and processing the vitamins became overwhelmed.

At the same time, the water-soluble vitamins were thought to be easily disposed of by your body. Take too many of the B vitamins, vitamin C, biotin, and pantothenic acid and supposedly your kidneys could eliminate them quickly and easily in your urine. This method of disposal led many vitamin naysayers to claim that taking vitamins didn't help your health; supplements merely gave you some of the most expensive urine in the world.

More recently, the dividing lines between which vitamins are supposed to be safe in large quantities and which are dangerous have been redrawn. The original, simple idea that water-soluble vitamins were invariably safer than the fat-soluble nutrients turned out to be too simplistic. For instance, niacin, one of the water-soluble vitamins, can be very dangerous when taken in large doses. And when niacin is given to heart disease patients in an effort to control levels of the blood fats called triglycerides, there is a danger of liver damage. That is why doctors who prescribe pharmacological doses of this nutrient must frequently do blood tests to make sure liver function is not compromised.

The safety of taking vitamin E in relatively large doses also runs counter to the conventional wisdom. Some older books would have you believe that this fat-soluble vitamin is dangerous in daily quantities over 100 IU, but it has been shown to be extremely safe in quantities up to and over 800 IU a day.

Vitamin E Units

The exact definition of an international unit of vitamin E is rather technical since there are many different types of tocopherol that are considered forms of vitamin E. Alpha-tocopherol, the most useful for the body and the most plentiful in food, is rarely available in pure form in vitamin supplements. When this nutrient is synethesized in the lab or vitamin factory, it emerges mixed up with what are called stereoisomers, molecules that are chemically similar to alpha-tocopherol but not quite the real thing. If you look at vitamin jars closely, you'll find that natural vitamin E or natural alpha-tocopherol (this is the tocopherol without the stereoisomers) is often designated d-alpha-tocopherol, while synthetic vitamin E is frequently listed as dl-alpha-tocopherol. The more up-to-date but equally confusing designation of natural vitamin

E is supposed to be RRR-alpha-tocopherol, while the synthetic should be called all-rac-alpha-tocopherol.

The international unit is defined as vitamin E that has the biological activity of one milligram of the synthetic acetate of all-rac-alpha-tocopherol. The important number to remember is that the RDA for vitamin E for adults is 10 IU for men and 8 IU for women.

Many nutrition researchers are taking much more of this vitamin—as much as 800 IU a day—because of its apparent benefits.

Fortunately, this vitamin is considered very safe, even when taken in ridiculously large amounts. The only vitamin takers who may have been consistently overdosed on this vitamin appear to be some premature infants who were injected with large doses in an effort to prevent the eye damage that can be caused by the oxygen therapy they frequently undergo.

Despite some scare stories of vitamin E causing fatigue, high blood pressure, and creatinuria, these symptoms have not been observed in reliable scientific studies. In fact, the most often reported side effect is a stomachache, and even that symptom is relatively rare.

For instance, in a series of studies in which people took from 600 to 3,200 IU of vitamin E a day, there were no significant side effects reported. However, most experts recommend that vitamin takers keep their daily dose down to 800 IU or less. Some advocate taking anywhere from 200 to 600 units a day.

One caveat: If you are taking an anticoagulant drug such as Wafarin or have a vitamin K deficiency, you should discuss vitamin E with your doctor before taking supplements. Since vitamin E can make your blood take longer to clot as do anticoagulant drugs, taking the vitamin at the same time may promote the formation of hemorrhages. A vitamin K deficiency may also have the same effect.

Of course, if you are taking any kind of medication, talk to your doctor before taking vitamin supplements.

9

Vitamin K

Vitamin K is an important nutrient since your blood could not clot without it, but its importance as a part of the diet or as a supplement is limited for adults. The bacteria in our intestines can manufacture this family of related compounds that we refer to as vitamin K.

Vitamin K was originally discovered in chickens. A researcher in Copenhagen fed chicks a fat-free diet and found that it caused them to develop a hemorrhagic disease: Their blood refused to coagulate. Consequently, he termed the nutrient *koagulationsvitamin*, a Swedish tongue twister that refers to its coagulating function in the body. In any language, it's easier to refer to this substance as vitamin K.

Adults don't need to consume much vitamin K. Their bodies can both store and produce their own reserves of this nutrient. However, newborn babies, who don't have a supply of the intestinal bacteria that makes vitamin K, sometimes develop hemorrhagic disease unless they receive vitamin K supplementation after being born. Doctors usually give newborns a shot of it to make sure they have an adequate supply until the bacteria in their intestines bloom.

Other than in babies, vitamin K deficiency is rare and usually only occurs in people who are on antibiotics for a long time. These drugs can kill off the intestinal bacteria that supply much of our vitamin K. In cases like those, anyone suspecting they are suffering vitamin K deficiency should consult their doctor.

Most of Us Make All the Vitamin K We Need

Occasionally, people with heart disease who are taking blood thinners to slow blood clotting are also given vitamin K to partially offset the anticlotting properties of their drugs. The only other people who usually need vitamin K are the severely malnourished or those who have serious problems digesting the fat from their diet, since this is a fat-soluble vitamin. In those cases, the lack of nutrients entering the body from the digestive tract interferes with the movement of vitamin K from the liver into the bloodstream.

Most adults will never need vitamin K supplements. In the diet, this nutrient is found in leafy green vegetables as well as in egg yolks, liver, tomatoes, and cheese.

Taking vitamin K supplements probably won't help you, but it probably won't hurt you, unless you are taking blood thinners. In that case, always consult with your doctor before you take any vitamin supplements.

Even though vitamin K is a fat-soluble vitamin, and, according to the old wisdom, fat-soluble vitamins are stored longer in the body and are supposed to be more dangerous than water-soluble vitamins, large doses of this nutrient are not considered dangerous. Overdoses of vitamin K resulting in injury have not been reported. If you take a megadose, which is not recommended, your body will merely eliminate it in your urine, and your intestines will keep making more.

10

Setting Up Your
Optimal Health Plan

As should be evident from the information in this book, drawing up an optimal health plan for yourself involves more than just analyzing your nutritive needs and planning a program of vitamin supplementation. You also should follow a consistent exercise program and eat a low-fat diet. In addition, for optimal health, you should learn how to deal with stress, but that is beyond the scope of this book. Vitamin supplementation has to fit into an overall health scheme that is integrated into your total lifestyle. Within that context, vitamin supplements should play an important role in your optimal health plan.

You also have to decide what optimal health means to you. This is not always easy. A personal definition of optimal health is many faceted. Optimal health usually includes feeling your best, being free of disease, and possessing large stores of personal energy. To some, it's being able to meet athletic challenges such as running marathons. To others, it is primarily performing up to full capacity at work.

In searching for ways to build up their bodies and minds toward optimal health, many people find that day-to-day living tears them down rather than furthering their wellness goals. Stressful jobs deplete mental reserves, healthy foods are often scarce at business lunches, and busy schedules make it hard to find time to relax, exercise, or deal with stress via meditation or other methods.

Another impediment to constructing an optimal health plan is the babble of advice that constantly flows from the media. Newspaper columnists, celebrities, television announcers, and magazine writers, to name a few, claim to be able to tell us how to run our lives. They tell us where to invest our money, what clothes to wear, how to exercise, and what to eat.

In fact, in the cacophony of advice, the endless stream of instruction that comes out of the nutrition and vitamin field may be the most confusing of all. When it comes to what foods and vitamins you should incorporate in your optimal health plan, there is no shortage of experts claiming to know what's best. The trouble is, much of their advice is confusing, contradictory, based on little more than guesswork, and sometimes it is just plain idiotic.

Spotlight on Nutrition

The most reliable nutrition advice should have well-established scientific evidence to back it up. The backbone of a scientific field like nutrition is the definitive research upon which our knowledge of nutrition is supposed to rest. Carefully constructed experiments objectively test how humans and animals react to the consumption of individual nutrients. These experiments are augmented with epidemiological studies that compare the diets of various populations with the diseases those populations contract.

Years ago, almost all scientific studies were carried on in obscurity. In those days, when scientists published their studies in arcane journals, to be read only by other scientists, little note was taken of them in the popular media unless the research had immediate, dramatic consequences for human health. A new vaccine for polio was a page-one headline, but research into the physiology of digestion would never penetrate the public's consciousness.

All that changed when, sometime in the late 1960s and early 1970s, we became a nation intrigued with our health. Did I say intrigued? Obsessed would be a better word. As our life expectancy increased, and many infectious diseases were effectively quelled with antibiotics, we became less concerned about diseases like pneumonia, tuberculosis, and measles and turned our attention to avoiding diseases like cancer and heart disease that modern medicine seemed unable to vanquish.

At this time, doctors and medical researchers were making progress in inventing better ways to treat heart disease and cancer, but they seemed unable to devise methods for preventing these conditions. Coincidentally, a few out-of-the-mainstream nutrition scientists began to promise that where medical science had failed at preventive medicine, they had succeeded. All you had to do was eat a few beneficial foods, and/or take specific nutrient supplements, and long life and better health would be yours.

Frustrated with conventional medicine's lack of progress against the twin killers heart disease and cancer, increasing numbers of people began to buy books and magazines that promised to deliver super health through super diets. A few of these books became best-sellers. Simultaneously, subscriptions to health magazines climbed into the millions. Despite the hype and the promise of health benefits, many of the diets promoted by these books and magazines—in particular the weight loss programs such as the no-carbohydrate diets and the very low calorie diets—turned out to be dangerous. Almost all of these diets claimed to be based on scientific research, so, like it or not, scientific studies were thrown into the spotlight.

Around this same time, as soon as the editors and publishers of the mainstream media saw how popular health information had become, they began reporting on medical and nutrition studies that appeared in publications like the *Journal of the American Medical Association* and *The New England Journal of Medicine*.

We still have not recovered or adjusted well to this change in the reporting of scientific developments. All too often, preliminary studies are treated in the media as though their results were definitive. This is especially true when research can be turned into a health-scare story that makes juicy headlines.

Consequently, when follow-up studies show that the original research came to a mistaken conclusion, the public often grows confused and even angry at being misled. The result is cynicism toward a wide range of health information and the erroneous belief that research can show that any food or pleasurable activity is injurious to health.

Making Sense of Nutrition News

As a result of the constant reporting of scientific studies, many of which seem to contradict each other, it has grown much more difficult for consumers to know what health information to believe. Hyperbole infects much of the journalism that passes itself off as health reporting, and scant attention is paid to the real significance, or lack of significance, of the studies that make the news. However, there are some simple things you should look for when trying to decide how to interpret and put to use reports of alleged vitamin, nutrition, and health discoveries.

First of all, find out if the new research has been conducted at a reputable institution and if it was reported in a well-known medical journal (these include *Lancet, Nature, The New England Journal of Medicine,* the *Journal of the American Medical Association,* as well as others). The stature of the institution doing the research and the journal recording it is not always an indication of the research's reliability, but it does indicate how seriously the medical establishment will take it.

In theory, at least, research that has been funded by a government agency such as the Center for Disease Control in Atlanta, and subject to several layers of bureaucratic review may be more reliable than research performed in an independent lab that didn't qualify for government money. While some experts think that these experiments are often better constructed than other studies, government approval really reflects more the approval of the establishment than any innate scientific worthiness.

On the other hand, if a company or industry funds studies that support their vested interests, it is a good idea to take their results with the proverbial grain of salt. There are many cases of these kinds of findings: Much of the research in the 1980s showing that oats are beneficial to serum cholesterol was funded by manufacturers of oatmeal. Similarly, research showing that walnuts are good for your cardiovascular system was funded by the California Walnut Commission. Some of the studies demonstrating the heart healthy benefits of polyunsatured fats were funded by margarine manufacturers. Studies showing that bald men had increased risk of heart attack was paid for by Upjohn, a pharmaceutical manufacturer who produces a medicine that makes hair grow.

In each of these cases, the research may have been valid, but the conclusions can be skewed to the benefit of the funding corporation: Oats lower cholesterol, but it's the soluble fiber in oats that do the job, and soluble fiber is found in a wide range of fruits and vegetables, not just oats. As for walnuts, these nuts may be good for you, but equally beneficial are peanuts, cashews, and other nuts.

A little more insidious is the publicity given polyunsaturated fats. These fats are better for your heart than saturated fats, but the polyunsaturates in margarine that are hydrogenated (they have hydrogen added) may be harmful.

As for the bald men in the Upjohn study, Upjohn was trying to prove that patients taking their medicine were getting heart attacks because they were bald, not because they were applying the Upjohn product Rogaine (minoxidil). The scientific jury is still out on whether or not Upjohn proved its point.

A point to remember is that much of the research showing the benefits of vitamins is funded by—you guessed it—the vitamin manufacturers. That doesn't disprove the value of the research. Much of it is unassailable. But it should make you look closer at the conclusions to make sure that these studies really prove what they claim to prove.

Testing Research Reliability

One of the standard scientific means for testing the veracity of research is whether or not the test results can be replicated by other researchers performing identical experiments. In other words, if a researcher in Oregon finds that a certain vitamin cures ingrown toenails in thousands of people and then another researcher in

Alabama gets the same results using the same vitamin on thousands of other people, the research findings are generally considered to be dependable.

What often happens in nutrition and medical research, however, is that a few scientists will conduct similar experiments with nutrients and some of the researchers will produce a specific result while others will get a quite different outcome.

In the real world, it is rare that a group of researchers, even when they are accomplished scientists performing identical experiments, emerge with identical results. Hidden variables among the test subjects and other factors can skew test findings. Usually, in cases where a large majority of scientists get a specific result while only a few experimenters disagree, the majority rules. Whatever outcome most of the researchers found is deemed the acceptable answer unless somebody thinks of some serious reason to doubt that conclusion.

Researchers who found unsubstantiated results often use statistics to explain why their results weren't valid or various theories are conjured up to figure out why their experiments didn't jibe with the expected outcomes.

In many cases, the most widely accepted nutritional facts are those that have been replicated many times by reputable researchers. If your morning paper trumpets some new study that presents a totally unexpected result, you may be impressed, but most experienced scientists will want to see several studies confirming the result before they believe its conclusions.

Cause and Effect

If you go beyond the headlines and glib summaries of much of the research that gets reported in the popular media, you will often find that the concrete results of some studies may not be precisely the conclusions you hear about on the evening news. This is especially true with research that doesn't test substances in a lab but uses surveys to try to find out what circumstances are associated with illness. For example, reports on research into heart disease recently claimed that most heart attacks occur right after you get up early in the morning. What those researchers did was simply go over hospital records and check the time that heart attacks were recorded. From the way this study was reported in the media, you might think that a good way to avoid heart disease would be to simply sleep late. What the research really demonstrated is that the risk of heart attack peaks an hour after rising, no matter what time you climb out of bed.

Another caveat for health consumers is the necessity to watch out for superficial reporting of vitamin research. As you will note in this book, I constantly emphasize the need to combine a healthy diet that contains many vegetarian foods with any kind of vitamin supplemention program you implement. Despite the fact that supplements may be able to improve your health, diet is of paramount importance to an optimal health plan. Here again, a close look at the nutrition research behind the headlines confirms this: Most of the studies that support the health benefits of particular vitamins consist of research that examines the foods people eat, not merely the supplements they take.

When the newspapers report that antioxidants like beta-carotene have been found to help fight cancer and heart disease, usually it means researchers found that healthy people ate more fruits and vegetables rich in beta-carotene than did sick people, not necessarily that they were taking beta-carotene pills.

Of course, this is not always the case. Most notably, surveys of vitamin C status found that those who take vitamin C lived longer and enjoyed other benefits over those who generally didn't take supplements. In addition, other surveys have found that pregnant women who took multivitamins gave birth to fewer babies with birth defects. There have been many other studies that primarily focused on the use of supplements for health.

As each new survey about nutrition and vitamins is reported in the mainstream press, be sure and note whether the researchers were studying the pure vitamin in the lab, examining the health of those who took supplements, or whether they were looking at people who ate foods containing the vitamin.

Guilt by Association

Many of the larger population studies that give birth to headlines and magazine pieces on health are constructed from the associations researchers make between particular diseases and the health habits seemingly prevalent among people who come down with those diseases. For instance, the earliest studies that compared fiber consumption in Africa and in Europe and the United States found an association between the eating of refined, nonfibrous foods with diverticulitis and other digestive disorders (see page 233). At the same time, eating a high-fiber diet was associated with fewer incidences of these conditions.

What's important to remember when noting the results of studies like this is that the association of a disease with a lifestyle factor such as dietary fiber does not prove that the factor causes the disease the researchers are interested in. In this case, there is strong evidence to believe that fiber does have something to do with preventing diverticulitis. Other associations might not be as strong.

For instance, you could do a survey showing that as diverticulitis was increasing in the United States beginning in the 1950s, the sales of baseball cards also increased dramatically. Does that prove that baseball cards have a meaningful association with this disease? Probably not, even though Africans, whose digestive systems are often in better shape than ours, couldn't tell the difference between a Saint Louis Cardinal or a Colorado Rocky.

Care must be taken when interpreting associations derived from large-scale studies. For instance, research on women of childbearing age shows that those who take birth control pills are more likely to contract cervical cancer than diaphragm users. This association didn't show that birth control pills cause cancer but that diaphragms can stop a virus linked to cervical cancer.

Another study established that people who ingest greater quantities of the artificial sweeteners aspartame and saccharin weigh more than people who eat sugar. Again, this does not show cause and effect. The low-calorie, artificial sweeteners do not cause weight gain. On the contrary, the results of this research shows that overweight people are more likely to turn to these chemicals in an effort to lose weight. In other words, they already weighed more than average before they began using artificial sweeteners.

How High My Risk?

Although the media loves to play up the frightening scare stories that come out of medical and nutritional research, sometimes the worrisome articles you see in the paper overstate and misinterpret the risk that has been discovered. For example, you may have read of a study that found that women who took estrogen replacement therapy had an increased chance of developing certain types of cancers such as breast cancer and endometrial cancer.

While that sounds scary, it does not present a reason for older women to stop taking estrogen unless they have other significant risk factors for cancer. For, in fact, doctors know that estrogen replacement therapy also lowers women's risk of heart disease, a much more prevalent killer of postmenopausal women than cancer.

A way to ascertain the significant risks and benefits emerging from these studies is to look for articles describing how the researchers themselves have altered their lifestyles in reaction to their findings. Not long ago, Walter Willett, a Harvard professor who is involved in an ongoing study of the dietary habits of more than 100,000 nurses in what's known appropriately enough as The Nurses' Health Study, told the Los Angeles *Times* that the results of his research have led him to start taking vitamin E supplements. He has also given up red meat altogether because of its association with colon cancer. When an expert like Willett concedes the benefits of these measures, then you can rest assured that the lifestyle changes described are based on reliable observations.

The Real World of Vitamins

Remarkable as it seems, with all the nutritional research that has gone on in the past few years, much of the information available on vitamins is hearsay, rumor, and scientific guesswork. As Ralph Shangraw, a pharmaceutical professor at the University of Maryland, recently told the *Nutrition Action Healthletter,* "It's incredible how little we know about nutrient supplements."

One difficulty for consumers in finding out information about vitamins and nutrition is that few experts in the field are completely objective. Some are paid consultants to pharmaceutical companies, vitamin manufacturers, or food companies. Others have pet theories that they promote. For instance, as we've mentioned, several years ago when oats were being heralded as cholesterol-lowering because of their soluble fiber content, not many people recognized that the scientific studies supporting this benefit were sponsored by food companies with large investments in oat cereals. Accompanying the research was a barrage of public relations efforts, once again paid for by food companies, who wanted to make sure the world knew that oats could lower cholesterol. Left out in all the hoopla was the fact that although a modicum of oats may be good for you, no one knows the long-term effects of consuming bowl after bowl of oatmeal to the neglect of other fibrous foods.

The vitamin field is filled with similarly misleading statements, many of which are technically true but omit more than you might be aware of. The claims of many of the vitamin companies that their products meet the highest standards of purity are a good example of this. Those claims are probably true, but the fact is, most of the vitamins inside vitamin jars are manufactured by a relatively few large companies who sell them in bulk to other companies who wholesale them to retail stores. The raw ingredients distributed among the various vitamin brands is fairly homogeneous. Mostly what is unique from brand to brand are the labels and bottles.

In some ways, buying vitamins is a bit like buying gasoline. Gasoline retailers frequently buy their wares in bulk from wholesalers. Although different gas stations fly different flags, display different brand names, and sport various little animals and logos, high-test and regular at one brand-name station may have come from the same supply as the gas at the competing station across the street.

In the same way, the ingredients inside one fancily decorated vitamin jar may have come from the same source as the drab, house-brand bottle sitting next to it on a pharmacy shelf. If you are economy minded, you can usually stick to the house brand and be confident that you are not shortchanging yourself. According to the Center for Science in the Public Interest (CSPI), a consumer-watchdog group based in Washington, D.C., you can assure yourself of quality vitamins by buying store brands from retailers with well-developed national reputations. These chains have vitamin quality executives who keep a close eye on the vitamins sold to them by manufacturers.

Vitamin Formulations

Of course, despite the proliferation of gasoline brand names, picking out the right octane gas for your car is a lot easier than buying the right vitamin formula for your body. Gas stations mostly limit their gas selection to regular, high-test, and something in between. Vitamin companies, in contrast, have combined their ingredients in enough different mixtures to fill an encyclopedia (or a pharmacy shelf or two).

Because vitamins are classified as foods, there are few restrictions on the combinations of nutrients that are allowed to be put into vitamin formulas. Most of the federal restrictions are on the quantity of minerals allowed since minerals pose greater health risks than vitamins. In addition, the Food and Drug Administration limits the folate content of vitamins to 400 milligrams. Occasionally, megadoses of folate can mask but not cure pernicious anemia, a vitamin B_{12} deficiency (see page 67).

The vitamin formulas that companies have come up with are usually arbitrary or may be based on marketing surveys and the cost of raw ingredients. Since many of the B vitamins are cheap to produce, multivitamins frequently contain large amounts of these nutrients. Other ingredients that are more expensive, such as biotin, are generally inserted in much smaller amounts.

Sometimes, vitamin companies seem to produce supplements in certain proportions for no reason at all other than the fact that they've always done it the same way. When CSPI contacted a vitamin company that bragged its formulas were "based on clear scientific evidence rather than the fad of the moment" and asked for an explanation for the proportions of vitamins found in one of its products, the company was unable to present a meaningful rationale. It was a formula the company had produced for more than twenty years. It still sold well. That seemed to be reason enough to keep making it.

The Problem With Natural

A favorite word of vitamin companies as well as food companies, manufacturers, and cosmetic companies is the adjective *natural*. Since the word is so popular among consumers, it is emblazoned on everything from vitamins to cookies to face cream in an effort to boost sales.

What this word really does in most cases is boost confusion, since there is no generally accepted definition of natural, and even when experts do agree on what it means, the word is not always very helpful in discerning vitamins or other products that are better for you than their artificial competitors.

The problem with attaching the description to vitamins is the difficulty of calling anything natural that is processed and refined enough to stick into a little pill or capsule. In their normal natural habitat, vitamins are present in food, accompanied by a vast array of other chemicals that are taken out when the vitamin is made into pill form. Calling a vacuum-packed bottle of vitamins natural is like calling a lion in a zoo natural. No matter how appealing the zoo grounds appear, a zoo is not an animal's normal living space, and a jar is not a vitamin's normal environment.

In general, the only vitamin some experts believe is better utilized in its so-called natural form is vitamin E, whose most active natural formulation is noted on vitamin jars as d-alpha-tocopherol.

The Many Steps in Making a Natural Vitamin

But even with natural vitamin E, the complexities involved in vitamin extraction don't really allow any unrefined products to be packaged in pill or capsule form. According to Paul Huff, reporting in the *Journal of Applied Nutrition,* getting vitamin E out of the soybean, the most commonly used raw material, involves more than seven difficult chemical steps.

To prepare the raw material of vitamin E for extraction, it is first soaked in a hot solution of caustic soda. Then hexane is used to take out the crude vegetable oil from the soybean. After the oil is filtered (at a pressure of 50 pounds) material that is insoluble is taken out and the hexane is evaporated and recycled.

The oily mixture that results is opaque and possesses unpleasant odors and taste. This mixture is heated and treated with nitrogen and other gases before hydrochloric acid and methanol are added to separate the sludge from the rest of the clear, odorless oil.

At this point, with the acid and methanol removed, the oil may be bottled and sold as cooking oil, but the sludge has to be further processed to make natural vitamin E. These extra processing steps include cooling and further filtering to remove sterols (chemicals that can be used as synthetic hormones), washing with water to take out substances such as inositol, choline, and glycerol, vaccuum distillation that removes fatty acids, washing and filtering with methanol to take out more sterols and other undesirable material, and then removal of the remaining methanol via distillation.

Then the final product, a mixture of tocopherols (forms of vitamin E), is finally ready for insertion into a capsule. This capsule, despite the many layers of processing that have gone into its ingredients, can then be labeled natural vitamin E.

Dissolving Vitamins

Arguments have raged about how well vitamin and mineral pills dissolve in the digestive tract, causing some experts to question how much of the vitamins you swallow in pill form actually make it into your blood. Since supplements are worthless if they pass through you without breaking down and being taken in by the body, researchers have been disappointed to find that calcium tablets and some other preparations took a long time to dissolve, throwing doubt on their usefulness. At one point, in the 1980s, it was found that about one out of two calcium supplements took more than half an hour to dissolve when subjected to a laboratory test that simulated conditions in the stomach.

At the same time, CSPI reported that Dr. Shangraw tested various multivitamins and found that almost half of the pills he tested took more than two hours to dissolve, much too long to be sure that they would be absorbed adequately into the bloodstream.

According to Dr. Shangraw, the problems with the calcium pills could have arisen from the compression of the nutrients. They were pressed together too firmly in order to make a smaller pill that was easier to swallow. In addition, their coating with shellac (considered a natural ingredient) resisted dissolution by stomach acid, plus the cementlike gelatin used to hold them together and the lack of starch in the supplements limited absorption.

Luckily, vitamin and mineral supplements in the future should break down a little more quickly. The U.S. Pharmacopoeia Convention (USP), a scientific group chartered by Congress with the responsibility for setting and maintaining drug composition standards, has now moved toward setting standards for the disintegration of supplements. As of January 1993, the USP standard for formulations containing the water-soluble vitamins (the B complex vitamins, vitamin C, biotin, and pantothenic acid) will require that uncoated vitamin pills disintegrate in thirty minutes or less in the standard lab test. Coated vitamins will be required to break up in forty-five minutes or less.

Although the USP standard is not mandatory, it is hoped that competitive pressure will force most companies to comply with these standards. If they do, it should be noted on the label. Alternatively, some vitamin companies have begun listing dissolution times on their labels. This information explains how long the vitamin pills take to dissolve in the digestive tract fluids. It is considered very desirable if a supplement dissolves in less than forty-five minutes, since dissolution of a vitamin occurs after disintegration and is one step closer to absorption through the walls of the stomach and intestines.

Along with its standards for water-soluble vitamins, in the future the USP plans to come up with disintegration standards for the fat-soluble vitamins (vitamins A, D, E, and K) as well as requirements for multivitamins, minerals, time-release formulas, and chewable pills.

If you purchase vitamins whose labels have no data about dissolution time or compliance with the USP standards, you still may be able to discover this for yourself. Many labels include a customer service phone number where you can reach a company representative who should have access to this information.

Expiration Dates

Just as cereals, milk, juice, and just about everything else in the supermarket list the last dates they are supposed to be available for sale, most vitamins now also list expiration dates. Milk companies fairly consistently base their dates on the time they believe milk stays fresh, and bread bakers have a good idea about the shelf life of their loaves, but vitamin manufacturers base their dates on—well, the truth is, no one knows.

Until recently, few vitamins carried expiration dates, but consumers got so used to seeing these dates everywhere that vitamin companies decided to give consumers what they wanted. It's as though they said, "You want expiration dates? We'll give you expiration dates." The rationale for these dates is elusive, since large-scale studies of how long vitamins keep their potency have not been carried out. Apparently, the vitamin companies just make their best guess and stamp it on the vitamin jar. The world of prescription drugs, as you may have guessed, is a lot more tightly regulated. Drug expiration dates have to be based on tests of chemical stability.

Despite the unreliability and arbitrariness of vitamin expiration dates, consumer groups like CSPI insist you check these dates and avoid bottles whose dates are within nine months of expiring. Their reasoning seems to be that if the printed expiration date is about to arrive, the vitamins in the jar must be at least several years old. I can't find any reason to argue about that, but don't take these dates too seriously until someone comes up with some verifiable standards.

Vitamin Additives

How worried should you be about the other ingredients—the additives—that are put into your vitamin pill along with the nutrients? Even though many vitamin jars headline the fact that they are virtuously starch- and sugar-free, these two ingredients actually help the digestive tract process the vitamins so they can be absorbed. Another reason for the addition of small amounts of sugar is to make chewable tablets and some mineral preparations more palatable.

There is a limit to how natural and free of additives a vitamin can be. After all, we are talking about the creation of a pill which has no obvious resemblance to anything nature ever created. If you take a liquid supplement, you may find that preservatives have been added. It is reasonable to think that the presence of a small amount of preservative to protect the vitamins is probably better for you than degraded nutrients.

If you are a strict vegetarian, take note that CSPI reports that most vitamin capsules are made from gelatin, an animal product. Capsules manufactured from vegetarian ingredients are usually indicated on the label. They will usually cost a little more, too.

The Potency Crap Shoot

Since so many people take vitamin supplements, you might think that a government agency would be standing over the manufacturers' shoulders keeping an eye on what goes into these pills. You'd be wrong. While vitamin makers often test competitors' products to see how well they match up with label claims, they are the only ones doing any kind of consistent testing, and the results of these tests are not available to the public. No government agency is making sure that vitamins contain what the jars say should be in them.

Vitamin makers argue that the present system works just fine, and the standards they have imposed on themselves are quite adequate. However, there are plans in the works for USP to set some potency standards to go along with new disintegration standards for vitamins. These may take years to work out and compliance with USP standards will be voluntary, not compulsory. Here again, the hope is that if some vitamin makers advertise the fact that they meet USP standards (whatever they turn out to be) other vitamin makers will feel forced by competitive pressure to also meet these standards.

In the meantime, as I've noted before, the consensus is that if you stick to national brands or the store brands of national retailers with a good reputation, chances are your vitamins will be reasonably potent. Be warned, however, that in the past even large national distributors have recalled vitamins because their products were weaker than advertised.

A test of potency you can conduct yourself—purely subjective and of unknown reliability—is to ask yourself how your vitamins make you feel. Does one brand make you feel better than another? If it seems to, stick to the brand that seems to work best. Another technique to make sure that you are getting adequate supplementation is to take different brands of supplements on different days or mix and match brands. That way, if one of the brands of supplements you take is below par but the others are adequate, you won't be going for very long without the nutrients you want to take.

The Most Desirable Nutrients

When planning your supplements for optimal health, you should start with a multivitamin that supplies the RDA for all of the vitamins and, if you want to take extra portions of other nutrients, you should take the antioxidant vitamins E, C, and beta-carotene, which seem to have the most benefits in helping prevent cancer and heart disease.

When picking out a multivitamin, it is permissible to take a brand that you only have to take once a day, although you may absorb slightly more of the vitamins if you take a formulation of lower strength and swallow the pills twice or three times a day with meals or snacks.

While most people take their multivitamin in the morning, this may not be the best time to take it if you currently eat a very low-fat or no-fat breakfast. The fat-soluble vitamins are generally absorbed more efficiently in the presence of fat. Taking your multivitamin with dinner, which often contains more oil than breakfast, may help your body utilize these nutrients.

Of course, the need to eat a little fat with your fat-soluble vitamins should not be a signal to eat a large helping of fatty food. Stay away from highly saturated fats such as those in red meats. Fats in margarine are hydrogenated, which renders them similar in physio-logical effect to saturated fats. A little peanut butter on bread is sufficient to aid vitamin absorption (eat the kind without the added hydrogenated oils) or dip bread into a small amount of olive oil, which will also supply enough fat to enhance your fat-soluble vitamin intake.

Nutrient Selection

One of the latest marketing ploys in the labeling of multivitamins is to announce the presence of beta-carotene among the ingredients. A barrage of publicity has established the health-enhancing characteristics of beta-carotene in the minds of vitamin consumers, so marketers have made sure that no matter how much or how little beta-carotene is in their product, the label prominently displays the fact that they have squeezed some of this nutrient into the pills.

You do want beta-carotene in your multivitamin supplement. As noted previously (see page 118) beta-carotene has a dual role in the body as a vitamin A precursor and as an antioxidant in its own right. Since vitamin A is of more limited usefulness and can be toxic in high doses when taken for a prolonged period of time, unlike beta-carotene, which only poses a possible danger if you drink large amounts of alcoholic beverages, it is preferable to take beta-carotene rather than other forms of vitamin A.

Because beta-carotene is often listed on the label along with vitamin A palmitate, fish oil, and vitamin A acetate as part of the vitamin A contents of the multivitamin, it isn't always possible to tell how much of the vitamin A is actually in the form of beta-carotene. You should look for multivitamins that break down these ingredients separately and list the majority of the vitamin A as beta-carotene. Ideally, all of the vitamin A should be beta-carotene, but if you buy a supplement that has a mixture of different types of vitamin A, make sure the non-beta-carotene vitamin A content is 5,000 IU or less. This is of special importance for women of childbearing age: Megadoses of vitamin A much above the USRDA of 5,000 IU can cause birth defects while beta-carotene does not have this toxic effect.

Multiple Ingredients

Along with the beta-carotene in your multivitamin, it's particularly important that your vitamin pill contain the RDA for folate. This nutrient is crucial for women of childbearing age since it may prevent birth defects. Just make sure that your multivitamin doesn't go very much over the RDA of 400 micrograms. CSPI thinks it shouldn't go beyond 600 micrograms for anyone. That's because folate can mask pernicious anemia, a vitamin B_{12} deficiency. If you develop this condition and take folate, some of the symptoms of anemia such as fatigue may lessen, but hidden nerve damage may still result as the pernicious anemia progresses. Of course, if you have any reason to suspect that you are suffering from anemia, see a doctor.

Is it worth having extra helpings of the antioxidants C and E in your multivitamin? Probably not. You can take these nutrients in separate pills that do not cost very much, while multivitamins containing substantial amounts of these nutrients are fairly expensive. It may be a good idea to take some extra beta-carotene as well, since all three of these nutrients are thought to work together to help prevent cancer and heart disease.

In any case, vitamin C rarely causes side effects at daily dosages from 200 milligrams to 1,000 milligrams. The most common problem you may have is loose stools, but some vitamin C advocates say you should take as much vitamin C as you can tolerate without developing diarrhea. Linus Pauling, the vitamin C booster emeritus who is in his nineties, takes about 18 grams (18,000 milligrams) a day of this nutrient. Even conservative nutrition experts say you should get at least 120 milligrams per day of vitamin C (this is twice the RDA) and then, if you come down with a cold, they recommend bumping up your daily dosage to about 1,000 milligrams to keep your cold symptoms in check and encourage them to go away. You probably won't find that large an amount in a multivitamin.

Vitamin E also probably won't be found in large amounts in many multivitamins. Researchers who have studied vitamin E recommend taking anywhere from 400 to 800 IU daily. Here, too, Linus Pauling advocates taking quite a bit. He swallows 800 IU of vitamin A supplements a day. A survey of doctors carried out by the *Medical Tribune* found that eight out of ten doctors answering their questionnaire tell their patients to take at least 100 IU of vitamin E a day.

Sufficient Nutrients

In contrast to the benefits of taking extra antioxidants, most experts are fairly unanimous in pooh-poohing the need for megadose helpings of vitamins B_1, B_2, and B_3, which are also known as thiamine, riboflavin, and niacin. However, if you exercise strenuously, a little extra of these nutrients, especially riboflavin, may help your body metabolize nutrients more efficiently when you work out. This is important for non–milk drinkers who exercise since milk is the chief dietary source for riboflavin. Otherwise, you only need the RDA for these nutrients.

You should also make sure that your multivitamin has at least but not more than 400 IU of vitamin D. This is crucial if you are elderly and do not get outside in the sun very much. Sunlight stimulates vitamin D production in the skin, but as you get older, your body becomes less efficient at producing this nutrient and, in the colder months, when you are all bundled up and the sun is low on the horizon, you may run a little short of this bone-enhancing chemical. Avoid megadoses of vitamin D. They can impair the function of your kidneys and cause other serious problems.

Where's the B_{12}?

If you have been cutting back on your meat consumption or if you have made the complete move to vegetarianism, make sure that your supplement contains the USRDA for vitamin B_{12}, a nutrient found only in meat, dairy products, and other foods made from animal sources. Lack of B_{12}, as noted above, can lead to pernicious anemia, a very serious condition that demands a doctor's attention. Some of the symptoms of anemia are weakness, pale skin, and shortness of breath.

Aside from vegetarians and those who hardly eat any meat or dairy products, the elderly may also need a little more of this vitamin. As you get older, the digestive system's ability to absorb B_{12} declines. Lack of this vitamin may cause mental confusion that can be mistaken for Alzheimer's disease.

Should There Be Minerals in Your Vitamins?

In most cases, your mineral needs are trickier to assess than your need for vitamins. The benefits of many minerals that are sold in supplements are unproven, and many of them that have been shown to be beneficial should only be ingested in very small amounts. Excess can result in more problems than a slight deficiency might cause.

If you decide to take minerals, pick out a multivitamin that does not have more than the USRDA for iron. Even though iron is necessary for the proper functioning of the immune system, a severe lack of iron is only a widespread problem in populations that suffer serious malnutrition. Most of us will not benefit from excess amounts.

As I point out in the section on iron (see page 208), the taking of large amounts of this mineral has made many nutrition experts uneasy because studies show that people with heart disease and cancer often display elevated iron levels. Whether or not taking iron supplements can actually cause these diseases or be a factor in their development has not been established.

Adult men and women after the age of menopause usually do not need extra iron except if they suffer from some types of anemia. If you think you have anemia, see your doctor. Do not try to treat it yourself with nutrition supplements. In most cases, pregnant women, nursing mothers, and children who are growing rapidly are the only ones who may need iron supplements, and they should stick to the USRDA.

Keeping Up With Zinc

Zinc has also become a popular supplement. Because the prostate gland has more zinc in it than most other parts of the body, zinc supplements have been sold as beneficial for this organ. There's no evidence to support this benefit, but zinc is important because it plays a role in more than one hundred vital enzymes. If you take zinc, stick to the USRDA and make sure your multivitamin supplement also includes a little bit of copper, since zinc can interfere with your body's copper absorption and utilization. There is no USRDA for copper, but the estimated safe range is 1.5 to 3 milligrams a day for adults. Labels on vitamin jars may mistakenly refer to amounts in this range as the USRDA. Avoid any supplement with more than this amount of copper, since this metal can act as an oxidant.

Selenium, Chromium, and Boron

When taking supplements that include minerals, your pills should include selenium and chromium but exclude boron or only include it in very small quantities. Selenium is an antioxidant that interacts with vitamin E to keep free radicals from damaging cell structures. Large amounts are toxic. They can make your hair fall out, give you bad breath, and do other unpleasant things to your appearance and health. The RDAs for selenium range between 55 and 70 micrograms for adults in good health. Your dosage should be in this range. CSPI recommends that you never exceed 200 micrograms a day.

Similar advice applies for chromium, a mineral that may be influential in preventing diabetes. The body uses chromium to keep blood sugar under control. According to the NRC, the estimated safe and adequate daily dietary intake for adults is about 200 micrograms. Do not exceed this amount.

The research on boron is just getting off the ground and there are no allowances for how much of this mineral you should ingest every day. In its report on trace elements whose roles are not well understood in the human body, the NRC reports that boron "appears to affect calcium and magnesium metabolism and may be needed for membrane function." Beyond that, researchers suspect that boron may influence the strength of your bones. Despite the fact that supplement makers have begun to sell boron in jars, it is not wise to take boron supplements. Too little has been reported on what a safe and effective intake of boron is.

Nobody's Minding the Store

If supplements like boron have not been proven to be safe, why are boron pills allowed to be sold as supplements? Shouldn't the Food and Drug Administration do something about this situation?

In theory, the FDA could step in and enforce strict rules on supplements, but it is not legally obligated to do so, and it will not, despite the fact that Americans spend more than three billion dollars a year on nutrients in jars. Those who head the agency feel they have their hands full dealing with the efficacy of drugs and problems with the food supply and that they do not have the resources to police supplements. As Dr. Kessler, the FDA head, told the *New York Times* about the FDA's attitude toward vitamin supplements, "We have not set any product standards, any manufacturing controls nor required any safety testing."

Much of the reason that the FDA stays outside of the supplement regulation business is in deference to the powerful political forces that prefer the situation the way it presently stands. Members of Congress, as well as the supplement makers and supplement taking members of the public have kept the FDA at bay, forestalling any efforts to keep a close eye on supplements. This prevents the agency from putting strict controls on what kinds of vitamin formulas can be sold. Otherwise, conservative regulators in the FDA might outlaw megadoses of some nutrients that are presently allowed.

It has been pointed out by many that if you wanted to sell cans of chicken noodle soup, you'd be more closely watched by the FDA than if you decided to become a vitamin marketer. To sell vitamins you do not need any kind of federal permits. All you need is the money to buy the raw product from a manufacturer, perhaps some licenses from the localities where you want to sell the supplements, and liability insurance in case an illness strikes your customers that they blame on your pills. In many cases, manufacturers will bottle your supplements for you, print up labels to your specifications, and set you up in business—for a price.

Just about the only time the FDA steps in to closely oversee supplements is when unsubstantiated health claims are made on the label or in the literature accompanying the nutrients. Even then, if the health claims are fairly benign, promising a little more pep, or other minor benefits, the FDA probably won't do anything. Only if the supplements claim to cure heart disease, cancer, AIDS, or some other really big disease, will the agency sit up and take notice.

Because of the FDA's sensitivity to health claims on labels, vitamin makers have adopted a labeling trick that many food manufacturers have long used. Instead of coming right out and making health claims, they put a name on the product that implies a health benefit that is otherwise never overtly stated. Anyone browsing the pharmacy shelves is sure to know what supplements tagged with monikers like Stressbusters, Musclemaker, Super Performance Formula, and Megafitness Tabs are supposed to do. Even if the rest of the label is innocuous and within the letter—if not the spirit—of the law.

Many in the nutrition field hope that these types of misleading names will be outlawed someday. But if the FDA ever does try to rein in names, you can be sure that decades of legal wrangling will ensue as supplement makers resist.

11

Quick Guide to the Vitamins

Fat-Soluble Vitamins

Fat-soluble vitamins are stored in human body fat and are generally not eliminated in the urine as efficiently as are the water-soluble vitamins. Therefore, these nutrients can generally be stored for longer periods of time.

While it used to be thought that it was dangerous to take large amounts of fat-soluble vitamins because they could build up to toxic levels in your body, this idea has been disputed. Currently, it is generally accepted that the vitamins A and D present the only serious risk of vitamin toxicity when taken in large doses over a long period of time. A few experts such as Dr. Linus Pauling argue that vitamin A can usually be taken in large doses without ill effects. However, it is not recommended taking more than twice the Recommended Daily Amount (RDA) specified by the National Research Council for vitamin A, and a dose equal to the RDA is probably safer. Liver damage is the most serious of the physiological problems blamed on large doses of vitamin A.

Vitamin D should not be taken in daily doses larger than the RDA. Special care should be taken when giving this vitamin to children because they usually receive adequate doses of vitamin D in fortified milk. Excess vitamin D may produce calcium deposits in the kidneys and other organs.

The fact that these vitamins are fat-soluble does not mean they contain fat. No vitamin contains fat or calories. Some studies have indicated that eating a small amount of fat at the same time as taking fat-soluble vitamins may help your body absorb these nutrients.

Vitamin A

Chemical Names: Retinol, retinaldehyde, retinoic acid, retinoids

Main Functions in the Body:

• Helps preserve night vision, present in the pigment in the eyes
• Maintains overall health of the eyes, keeps eyes lubricated
• Maintains resistance against respiratory infection
• Necessary for the health of the immune system
• Used in the maintenance of mucous membranes
• Helps in bone growth and good health of skin, teeth, and hair

Vitamin A Helps Protect Against:

• Cancer: Because vitamin A is toxic in large doses, its usefulness in treating cancer is limited.
• Infectious diseases: In areas of the world where vitamin A deficiency is rampant, diseases such as measles are frequently fatal.

Recommended Dietary Allowance:

Adult men: 1,000 retinol equivalents (RE) or about 3,300 IU

Adult women: 800 retinol equivalents or about 2,600 IU

Number of Americans who get less than the RDA: 50 percent

Number of Americans who get less than 70 percent of the RDA: 41 percent

Best Food Sources: Liver, fish liver oils, eggs, butter, cheese, fortified dairy products (milk). The body can covert carotenes present in carrots and other yellow-orange vegetables into vitamin A. It is estimated that about half of the vitamin A in your body is usually made from these sources. In older books, the carotenes (beta-carotene, alpha-carotene, and cryptoxanthin) are referred to as provitamin A.

Food Preparation Instructions: Avoid overcooking foods. Vitamin A absorption is enhanced in meals that also contain fat, protein, and vitamin E. Oxidized fats (for example, butter that has started to turn rancid) limits absorption.

Optimal Supplimentation: One or two times the RDA (up to about 2,000 RE or 10,000 IU a day)

• Do not take more than twice the RDA for this vitamin for an extended period of time.

• Vitamin A can be toxic in large doses. When very large doses of this vitamin have been given to pregnant women, it has caused birth defects.

• Use caution when taking multivitamins that contain vitamin A if you are also taking cod liver oil or fish oil capsules, which contain large amounts of vitamin A. The cumulative dose may be very large.

• The elderly may need extra vitamin A. As you get older, you may be more susceptible to conditions limiting your absorption and metabolic use of vitamin A.

Toxicity: Relatively high when taken in megadoses for an extended period of time. It can cause vomiting, headache, dryness of the mouth and other mucous membranes, liver damage, diplopia, alopecia, and abnormal bone formation. It can cause birth defects when taken by pregnant women.

Taking supplementary beta-carotene in large amounts is safer than taking vitamin A. The body can convert beta-carotene into vitamin A and safely discard the excess (see section on beta-carotene, page 118).

Vitamin E

Chemical Names: Tocopherols, tocotrienols

In supplements, natural vitamin E is designated d-alpha-tocopherol or RRR-alpha-tocopherol. Synthetic vitamin E is designated dl-alpha-tocopherol or all-rac-alpha-tocopherol.

Note: Of the substances that make up vitamin E, alpha-tocopherol is most efficiently absorbed and converted into a form the body can use.

Main Functions in the Body:

• Acts as an antioxidant that protects cellular structures from being damaged by free radicals
• Maintains health of the circulatory system, protects red blood cells from oxidative damage
• Preserves normal muscle function
• Boosts immunity by helping immune cells eliminate free radicals

Vitamin E Helps Protect Against:

• Heart disease: Helps prevent oxidation of cholesterol that is thought to lead to arteriosclerosis, may help prevent angina in those who already have heart disease, inhibits formation of blood clots

• Cancer: Prevents free radical damage to DNA and other cellular structures

• Cataracts: Low levels of vitamin E in blood associated with increased risk of cataracts

• Cigarette smoke and possibly other air pollutants: Vitamin E thought to defuse free radicals generated in lungs and other tissues exposed to air pollution

• Strokes: May lower risk of stroke

• Infectious diseases: Helps the body fight off colds and flu

• Muscle injuries resulting from exercise

• Neurological disorders: Protects neuron membranes from oxidative damage

Signs of Deficiency: Overt deficiency is rarely seen in humans except in serious diseases that limit fat and vitamin E absorption.

Recommended Dietary Allowance:

Adult men: 10 milligrams tocopherol equivalents or 10 IU

Adult women: 8 milligrams tocopherol equivalents or 8 IU

Number of Americans who get less than the RDA: N/A

Number of Americans who get less than 70 percent of the RDA: N/A

Best Food Sources: Wheat germ oil, vegetable oils, margarine, whole grains, nuts, green vegetables, whole grain cereals, egg yolks, liver

Food Preparation Instructions: Do not let vegetable oils turn rancid. The oxidation that causes rancidity destroys vitamin E.

Optimal Supplementation: Probably between 200 and 800 IU daily

• Although some nutritional experts are skeptical of the value of taking vitamin E supplements, and still trumpet the old claim that vitamin E is the vitamin looking for a disease, researchers who have investigated its antioxidant effects generally take up to 800 IU a day.

• The natural form of vitamin E (d-alpha-tocopherol) is absorbed more efficiently than the synthetic form (dl-alpha-tocopherol). Many vitamin E capsules are mixtures of both. Some proponents of vitamin E supplementation recommend taking capsules of natural tocopherol mixed with the other tocopherols.

• In experiments with victims of sickle cell anemia, researchers found benefit in giving subjects between 400 and 450 IU of vitamin E daily.

• Researchers investigating the ability of vitamin E to lower the risk of cataracts found that 400 IU daily reduced the risk of this eye disease.

Toxicity: Extremely low. Reports of vitamin E causing fatigue and creatinuria have not been substantiated in well-designed studies. Occasionally, vitamin E takers suffer upset stomachs, but this is an uncommon side effect.

• Heart disease patients who are taking anticoagulant drugs should not take large amounts of vitamin E. If this applies to you, consult your doctor before taking any vitamin supplements.

• If you are on a low-fat diet, you probably need vitamin E supplements since this vitamin will be lacking in the foods usually consumed in a low-fat diet.

Beta-Carotene and Other Carotenes

Chemical Names: Carotenoids, alpha-carotene, lutein, lycopene, beta-cryptoxanthin, canthaxanthin. Also referred to as provitamin A or vitamin A precursors

• Fruits and vegetables contain more than 500 different types of carotenes, many of which have not been studied in detail and have unknown benefits to human health. The five predominant carotenes found in our food are alpha-carotene, beta-carotene, beta-cryptoxanthin, lutein, and lycopene.

• Until recently, the carotenes were only considered important in their role as conversion material for vitamin A, but as antioxidants in the body—without being turned into vitamin A—they are now recognized as crucial to optimal health.

• To date, only beta-carotene is available in supplement form. The other carotenes must be eaten in food.

• Of the carotenes, beta-carotene is most efficiently absorbed and converted into vitamin A. Some carotenes, such as canthaxanthin, cannot be converted into vitamin A at all but are still believed to play a role as antioxidants in the body.

Main Functions in the Body:

• Acts as an antioxidant that protects cellular structures from being damaged by free radicals.

• Maintains health of the circulatory system, probably keeps cholesterol from being oxidized and converted to plaque that blocks blood vessels and causes arteriosclerosis. Studies show that people with high levels of beta-carotene in their blood have a lower risk of heart disease.

• Boosts immunity by helping immune cells eliminate free radicals. Researchers who gave beta-carotene to patients infected with the HIV virus found that the nutrient improved immune response and was associated with an increase in white blood cell count.

• Probably maintains the health of the eyes, which are exposed to frequent production of free radicals.

Carotenes Help Protect Against:

• Heart disease: Helps prevent oxidation of cholesterol that is thought to lead to arteriosclerosis. May help prevent angina in those who already have heart disease. Studies show that populations consuming large amounts of carotenes in fruits and vegetables have a lower risk of heart disease.

• Cancer: Prevents free radical damage to DNA and other cellular structures. Clinical research has shown beta-carotene may be able to reverse the progression of premalignant lesions. Carotenes also prevent cancer with nonoxidative functions, although this action has not been explained.

• Cigarette smoke and possibly other air pollutants: Smokers who have low levels of carotenes in their blood are more likely to develop cancer.

• Infectious diseases: Beta-carotene has been shown to bolster immunity. It works synergistically with vitamin E to defuse the destructive power of free radicals.

• Photosensitivity disorders: In people who are extremely sensitive to bright light (breaking out in rashes and hives), beta-carotene relieved symptoms in 80 percent of patients.

Signs of Deficiency: There is little or no research regarding overt deficiency of carotenoids.

Recommended Dietary Allowance:

Adult men: No RDA (Traditionally, carotene's significance in human nutrition has only been considered in light of its role as a precursor of vitamin A.)

Adult women: No RDA

Number of Americans who get less than the RDA: N/A

Number of Americans who get less than 70 percent of the RDA: N/A

Best Food Sources: Carrots, leafy green vegetables such as broccoli and kale, and winter squash are high in beta-carotene. Tomatoes and red peppers are low in beta-carotene but contain lycopene. Both spinach and cress are good sources of beta-carotene and lutein.

Food Preparation Instructions: Do not overcook vegetables. Steam vegetables with as little water as possible or microwave.

Optimal Supplementation: Between 15 milligrams and 50 milligrams per day of beta-carotene. Currently, of all the carotenes, only beta-carotene is available in supplement form.

• Research into the health benefits of the carotenes is relatively new, so not a lot is known about what dose or quantities are the most effective. In the past, the carotenes were only investigated in light of their conversion into vitamin A.

• Of the carotenes, beta-carotene has been studied the most, with researchers giving subjects up to 180 milligrams a day of beta-carotene without observing toxic effects. However, studies in animals have found that heavy consumption of alcoholic beverages combined with beta-carotene supplementation may cause liver damage.

• Studies in the United States are ongoing, testing the effectiveness of taking 50 milligram of beta-carotene every other day to prevent heart disease, strokes, and cancer. In Australia, doses of beta-carotene at 30 milligram a day are being tested for effect against cancer.

• To get an ample supply of all the carotenes, you should eat several servings of fruits and vegetables daily.

Toxicity: Extremely low. HIV patients have been treated with 180 milligrams a day of beta-carotene without toxic effect.

• The major side effect of taking large amounts of beta-carotene or eating a diet intensely rich in vegetables containing beta-carotene is an acquired yellow-orange hue in the face, hands, and feet. This is not considered to be dangerous. Cutting back on beta-carotene dosage makes the color fade.

• Smokers are probably beta-carotene deficient. They should probably take supplements and eat a primarily vegetarian diet of carotene-rich foods.

Vitamin D

Chemical Names: Calciferol, cholecalciferol

Main Functions in the Body:

• Helps the body absorb phosphorous and calcium from food
• Necessary for the proper formation and maintenance of bones and teeth
• Probably regulates many basic cell activities

Vitamin D Protects Against:

• Osteoporosis or osteomalacia: These conditions occur when insufficient calcium is deposited in bones, weakening them and making them vulnerable to breaking and bending. Vitamin D regulates the process of bone mineralization.
• Rickets: This is the condition in growing children caused by vitamin D deficiency. Bones are malformed and weak. Legs and backbone bend under the body's weight.

Signs of Deficiency: Increased risk of bone fractures, malformed bones

Recommended Dietary Allowance:

Adult men: 5 micrograms per day

Adult women: 5 micrograms per day

Number of Americans who get less than the RDA: N/A

Number of Americans who get less than 70 percent of the RDA: N/A

Best Food Sources: Fortified milk, fortified margarine, eggs, butter. The skin also forms this vitamin when exposed to sunlight.

Food Preparation Instructions: No special care is necessary. Vitamin D is not easily destroyed in food.

Optimal Supplementation: The RDA for this vitamin is sufficient. It is not safe to take large doses of vitamin D. In large amounts this vitamin may be very dangerous for young children, causing irreversible damage to the cardiovascular system and the kidneys. For healthy people, there is no evidence to show that more than the RDA is necessary for optimal health.

Toxicity: This vitamin can be dangerous in high doses leading to irreversible damage to the cardiovascular system and the kidneys. Some experts believe this substance should be classified as a hormone rather than a vitamin.

Vitamin K

Chemical Names: Phylloquinone, menadione

Main Functions in the Body:

- Helps the liver produce blood clotting factors
- Required for the synthesis of protein

• Required for proper formation of structures in the bones and kidneys

Vitamin K Protects Against:

• Hemorrhaging: The blood cannot clot properly without vitamin K. This is often a problem with newborns so they are given shots of vitamin K soon after birth.

Signs of Deficiency: Increased risk of bleeding and hemorrhaging

Deficiency of vitamin K hardly ever occurs except in newborns, those with a severe problem digesting and absorbing fat, hospital patients who are very ill and malnourished, and those taking antibiotics and other drugs for a long time.

Recommended Dietary Allowance:

Adult men: 80 micrograms per day

Adult women: 65 micrograms per day

Number of Americans who get less than the RDA: N/A

Number of Americans who get less than 70 percent of the RDA: N/A

Best Food Sources: Leafy green vegetables, dairy products, eggs, meats, cereals, and fruits. However, the exact amounts of vitamin K contained in foods has not been precisely measured.

Food Preparation Instructions: No special care is necessary.

Optimal Supplementation: The RDA for this vitamin is sufficient. For most healthy people, vitamin K is also produced by bacteria in the intestines. There is no evidence that vitamin K supplementation will aid optimal health.

Toxicity: For adults, this drug is safe in megadose amounts, although it is not recommended. However, it can be dangerous for newborns when administered in large amounts.

Anyone being treated with anticoagulant drugs should have their vitamin K status carefully monitored. If that applies to you, consult a physician.

Water-Soluble Vitamins

Even though most water-soluble vitamins are quickly and efficiently eliminated in the urine when taken in large doses that the body cannot utilize, taking megadoses of some of these nutrients can be harmful. In particular, large quantities of niacin and vitamin B_6 can be dangerous when taken without medical supervision. B_6 can cause nerve damage, and niacin can harm the liver. In contrast, vitamin C can be taken in relatively large doses without any apparent harm.

While the fat-soluble vitamins can be stored in your body fat, most water-soluble vitamins are not stored to any great degree. Therefore, you usually need to ingest some of these vitamins every day. In addition, water-soluble vitamins are more perishable than fat-soluble vitamins. To preserve these vitamins during food preparation, do not overcook vegetables and use as little water as possible during cooking. Steam or microwave your vegetables rather than boiling them.

Vitamin C

Chemical Name: Ascorbic acid

Main Functions in the Body:

• Used to make collagen, the main structural material of the body; preserves the health of gums, teeth, blood vessels, and bones.

• Acts as an antioxidant that keeps other antioxidants (such as vitamin E and beta-carotene) from being broken down by free radicals.

• When ingested with water contaminated by nitrates or meats preserved with nitrates or nitrites, it keeps carcinogens from forming in the stomach.

• Probably boosts immunity, since this nutrient is found in very high concentrations in immune cells. Immune cells often concentrate vitamin C up to a hundred times more densely than is found in the blood.

• Regenerates vitamin E. Research indicates that after vitamin E defuses harmful free radicals in the body, vitamin C probably helps recycle the vitamin E so that it can work against other destructive free radicals.

• Aids in the absorption of iron. When ingested at the same meal with vegetarian foods containing iron such as raisins, leafy green vegetables, and beans, vitamin C increases your iron absorption. However, it has no effect on the absorption of iron from meat.

Vitamin C Helps Protect Against:

• Heart disease: May keep serum cholesterol down and prevent high blood pressure, prevents oxidation of cholesterol that is thought to lead to arteriosclerosis

• Cancer: May prevent free radical damage to DNA and other cellular structures

• Common cold: Alleviates cold symptoms and shortens duration of the disease, but may not prevent colds

• Scurvy: Caused by a severe lack of vitamin C; characterized by bleeding gums, extreme fatigue and lethargy, loose teeth, pain in the muscles and joints, and sores that do not heal; generally only occurs in malnourished alcoholics and those on severely restricted diets

• Cigarette smoke and possibly other air pollutants: Inhaling cigarette smoke destroys the body's vitamin C. Studies show that smokers have reduced levels of vitamin C in their blood. The National Research Council believes that the vitamin C requirements for smokers are about twice as much as for nonsmokers

Signs of Deficiency: Bruises under the skin, bleeding gums, injuries and wounds heal slowly, possible lethargy and depression, painful joints, prolonged colds and infections

Recommended Dietary Allowance:

Adult men: 60 milligrams

Adult women: 60 milligrams

Number of Americans who get less than the RDA: 41 percent

Number of Americans who get less than 70 percent of the RDA: 26 percent

Best Food Sources: Citrus fruits (oranges, grapefruit, tangerines, lemons), strawberries, kiwi fruit, red and green peppers, broccoli, cauliflower, and red cabbage. Present in lower amounts in tomatoes and potatoes. Not found to any significant degree in meat or other animal products.

Food Preparation Instructions: Heat, light, and air destroy vitamin C. To preserve vitamin C content, do not cut vegetables or fruits far in advance of serving. Keep orange juice containers closed and in the refrigerator. Do not let them reach room temperature.

Optimal Supplementation: Very controversial

• Vitamin C proponents such as Dr. Linus Pauling advocate taking up to 18 grams a day (300 times the

RDA) of this nutrient. They also recommend taking the largest daily dose your system can handle without suffering diarrhea (in other words step up your daily dose until you reach your maximum without suffering loose bowels).

• Conservative nutrition researchers believe that the RDA, 60 milligrams a day, is sufficient for good health, but they recommend 120 milligrams a day for smokers. Only 10 milligrams a day are necessary to prevent the deficiency disease of scurvy.

• Experiments testing vitamin C's effectiveness against the common cold have given 500 to 1,000 milligrams a day to healthy subjects until they caught a cold and then have given them between 1,000 milligrams (1 gram) and 4,000 milligrams (4 grams) daily to fight cold symptoms. These amounts frequently curtailed the effects of colds and have often shortened the duration of the disease.

• Cancer researchers who have investigated ascorbic acid's effect on cancer prevention recommend taking 1,000 milligrams daily.

• Taking significant amounts of aspirin for arthritis or any other chronic condition increases your requirement for vitamin C.

• Smokers and heavy drinkers should take extra vitamin C. For optimal health, they should also quit smoking and drinking.

Toxicity: Extremely low. Although researchers used to think vitamin C megadoses caused kidney stones and other problems, these have not been substantiated. Large doses may cause loose, frequent bowel movements.

A much debated side effect attributed to the cessation of vitamin C supplementation is rebound scurvy. According to some nutrition scientists, if you take large daily doses of vitamin C and then abruptly stop megadosing, your body will have trouble adjusting and you will experience symptoms of scurvy such as bleeding gums and fatigue. Little reliable information is available regarding this alleged side effect associated with discontinuing vitamin C. To be safe, daily megadoses of vitamin C should be discontinued gradually. Cut down the dosage about 10 percent a day if you decide to stop ingesting large helpings of vitamin C.

If you never eat fresh fruits and vegetables, you usually need supplementation of vitamin C.

Vitamin B$_1$ (Thiamine)

Chemical Name: Thiamine pyrophosphate

Main Functions in the Body:

- Acts as a coenzyme that aids in the liberation of energy from carbohydrates
- Aids in the metabolism of certain amino acids
- Maintains health of the nervous system
- Maintains appetite
- Necessary for proper muscle tone

Thiamine Protects Against:
Beriberi: A thiamine deficiency disease characterized by depression, neurological disorders, malaise, decrease in appetite, and loss of muscle tone. In the United States, alcoholics are mainly at risk for beriberi.

Signs of Deficiency: Possible depression and mental confusion, leg cramps. Extreme deficiency is rare in the United States except among alcoholics and those eating a severely restricted diet. Elderly may have lower levels of thiamine.

Recommended Dietary Allowance:

Adult men: 1.5 milligrams per day

Adult women: 1 milligram per day

Number of Americans who get less than the RDA: 45 percent

Number of Americans who get less than 70 percent of the RDA: 17 percent

Best Food Sources: Meats such as pork and liver, whole grain and fortified cereals, peas, fortified pasta, wheat germ, oatmeal

Food Preparation Instructions: Do not overcook vegetables. Steam vegetables with as little water as possible or microwave. Avoid boiling vegetables; the water will drain off many of the B vitamins.

Optimal Supplementation: The RDA for this vitamin is probably sufficient. There is no evidence to show that more than the RDA is necessary for optimal health. Fevers and infections may raise the thiamine requirement.

Toxicity: Extremely low. The kidneys can easily eliminate excess amounts of this vitamin. Experimental subjects have been given 500 milligrams a day of thiamine without toxic effect.

Vitamin B$_2$ (Riboflavin)

Chemical Name: Riboflavin

Main Functions in the Body:

• Acts as a coenzyme that aids in the metabolism of carbohydrates, protein, and fat
• Maintains healthy skin

- Aids in healing cuts and wounds
- Maintains mucous membranes
- Interacts with vitamins B_6 and niacin in the production of the body's energy

Riboflavin Protects Against:
Skin problems, dermatitis, and anemia

Signs of Deficiency: Deficiency is rare in the United States. Signs include oral sores, anemia, painful cracks in the corners of the mouth, eye problems (especially sensitivity to light). Wounds and cuts will not heal adequately. People with poor appetites who do not each much, or are on very restricted diets may need riboflavin supplementation.

Recommended Dietary Allowance:

Adult men: 1.7 milligrams per day

Adult women: 1.3 milligrams per day

Number of Americans who get less than the RDA: 34 percent

Number of Americans who get less than 70 percent of the RDA: 12 percent

Best Food Sources: Dairy products, especially milk, are the most important source. Eggs, poultry, meat, fish, enriched and whole grains, leafy green vegetables, broccoli, asparagus, and brewer's yeast.

Food Preparation Instructions: Do not overcook vegetables. Steam vegetables with as little water as possible or microwave. Avoid boiling vegetables; the water will drain off many of the B vitamins. Do not buy milk in transparent containers since light will destroy its riboflavin content.

Optimal Supplementation: The RDA for this vitamin is probably sufficient for most people. There is no evidence to show that more than the RDA is necessary for optimal health. Exercise may increase your riboflavin requirement.

Toxicity: Extremely low. Researchers believe that your digestive tract is not capable of absorbing large enough amounts of this vitamin to hurt you.

Vitamin B₃ (Niacin)

Chemical Names: Nicotinic acid, nicotinamide, niacinamide

Main Functions in the Body:

- Acts as a coenzyme that aids in the metabolism of carbohydrates, protein, and fat
- Maintains healthy skin
- Interacts with riboflavin and vitamin B₆ in the production of the body's energy

Niacin Protects Against:

- Skin problems, dermatitis, and anemia
- Pellagra: A deficiency disease characterized by inflamed mucous membranes, diarrhea, dermatitis, and dementia
- High cholesterol: Niacin must be taken in very large amounts to benefit the cholesterol levels of your blood. Supplementation of niacin megadoses should only be performed under close medical supervision. Large doses of niacin can impair liver function and cause other illness

Signs of Deficiency: Deficiency is rare in the United States. Signs include skin rashes, irritability, diarrhea.

Recommended Dietary Allowance:

Adult men: 19 milligrams per day

Adult women: 15 milligrams per day

Number of Americans who get less than the RDA: N/A

Number of Americans who get less than 70 percent of the RDA: N/A

Best Food Sources: Meats, peanuts, fortified cereals and grains. Whole grains contain niacin in a form that the body cannot use efficiently. Milk and eggs contain tryptophan, an amino acid the body converts to niacin.

Food Preparation Instructions: Do not overcook vegetables. Steam vegetables with as little water as possible or microwave. Avoid boiling vegetables; the water will drain off many of the B vitamins. However, niacin survives cooking better than the other vitamins in the B complex.

Optimal Supplementation: The RDA for this vitamin is probably sufficient. For healthy people, there is no evidence to show that more than the RDA is necessary for optimal health. Taking large amounts of niacin to lower your cholesterol should only be done under a physician's supervision.

Although the human body can make niacin out of the amino acid tryptophan, you should never take tryptophan supplements. Currently, tryptophan supplements are banned in the United States since people taking this supplementhavedevelopedafrequentlyfatalblooddisorder.

Toxicity: This vitamin can be dangerous in high doses leading to liver damage. Large doses of some forms of niacin cause vascular dilation, expansion of blood vessels that cause a flushing feeling, usually in the face.

Vitamin B_6

Chemical Names: Pyridoxine, pyridoxal,
and pyridoxamine

Main Functions in the Body:

- Helps produce neurotransmitters that brain cells use to communicate
- Aids in the liberation of energy from protein
- Necessary for the synthesis of amino acids
- Necessary for the transportation of amino acids from cell to cell
- Interacts with riboflavin and niacin in the production of the body's energy
- Helps form the hemoglobin in red blood cells
- Necessary for the conversion of tryptophan (an amino acid) into niacin
- Stimulates fetal growth in pregnant women

Vitamin B_6 Protects Against:

- Anemia: B_6 is necessary for the proper formation of red blood cells.
- Nervous system disorders: The formation of chemicals involved in central nervous system function depends on vitamin B_6.
- Premenstrual syndrome: Symptoms may be alleviated. However, use of vitamin B_6 in this capacity is controversial and not universally accepted. Long-term use of large doses of vitamin B_6 may cause nerve damage. Do not use unless under close medical supervision.
- Carpal tunnel syndrome: Many doctors use this vitamin to treat pain in the thumb, wrist, and upper arm. This pain, which results from compression of the medial nerve that crosses the wrist, is often caused by prolonged repetitive motion such as typing or working on an assembly line. If you suffer carpal tunnel syndrome,

consult a doctor. In many cases vitamin B_6 has cured the pain. If it doesn't, surgery is frequently necessary to cure this condition.

Signs of Deficiency: Overt deficiency is rare in the United States. Signs include skin rashes, anemia, irritability, and diarrhea. In extreme cases, convulsions may occur.

Recommended Dietary Allowance:

Adult men: 2 milligrams per day

Adult women: 1.6 milligrams per day

Number of Americans who get less than the RDA: 80 percent

Number of Americans who get less than 70 percent of the RDA: 51 percent

Best Food Sources: Brown rice, whole wheat products, soybeans, oats, chicken, kidney, liver, fish, eggs, pork, peanuts, walnuts. Dairy products and red meats do not provide much of this nutrient.

Food Preparation Instructions: Do not overcook vegetables. Steam vegetables with as little water as possible or microwave. Avoid boiling vegetables; the water will drain off many of the B vitamins. Much of this vitamin is lost when vegetables are frozen or when cereals are refined (thus the necessity of eating whole grains).

Optimal Supplementation: The RDA for this vitamin is probably sufficient. For healthy people, there is no evidence to show that more than the RDA is necessary for optimal health. Taking large amounts of vitamin B_6 to combat premenstrual syndrome (PMS) can be dangerous and cause permanent nerve damage. Only do so under close medical supervision.

More than forty drugs have been shown to interfere with vitamin B_6 absorption and metabolism. If you have a chronic disease or are taking medications, consult your doctor about its interference with vitamin B_6. In many cases a supplement supplying the RDA may be necessary.

Taking oral contraceptives may interfere with vitamin B_6 metabolism. Women taking these contraceptives should take a multivitamin containing the RDA for B_6.

Pregnancy increases the need for vitamin B_6. Pregnant women should take a multivitamin supplement containing the RDA for B_6 and should consult a doctor.

Toxicity: This vitamin can be dangerous in high doses. Prolonged megadosing can cause nerve damage.

Folate

Chemical Names: Folic acid, folacin

Main Functions in the Body:

• Helps reproduce genetic material and helps make cell division possible
• Key ingredient in the process that produces hemoglobin in red blood cells
• Needed for periods of life when children grow rapidly
• Needed for protein synthesis

Folate Protects Against:

• Cancer: Folate may protect mucosal membranes from developing cancer. Preliminary studies of smokers with precancerous growths in their respiratory tract show that they have lower blood levels of folate than nonsmokers or smokers without these precancerous growths.
• Megaloblastic anemia: Folate is necessary for the adequate production of red blood cells. Megaloblastic

anemia is characterized by malformed red blood cells.

• Birth defects: Women who lack folate during pregnancy have an increased risk of giving birth to babies with spina bifida (a condition where the neural tube does not close properly) and other nervous system disorders. Incidences of babies born with cleft lips or palates may also be related to folate deficiency.

• Sprue: This gastrointestinal disease causes diarrhea, intestinal lesions, and problems absorbing nutrients from the digestive tract.

Signs of Deficiency: Overt deficiency is rare in the United States. However, pregnant women may be at special risk of damage to their unborn babies from a folate deficiency. Signs include fatigue and diarrhea.

Recommended Dietary Allowance:

Adult men: 200 micrograms per day

Adult women: 180 micrograms per day

Number of Americans who get less than the RDA: N/A

Number of Americans who get less than 70 percent of the RDA: N/A

Number of American women aged 19–50 who get less than 70 percent of the RDA: 87 percent

Best Food Sources: Leafy vegetables, yeast, liver, legumes (peanuts, lentils), oranges and orange juice, liver, kidney

Food Preparation Instructions: Folate is very sensitive to heat and light and can easily be destroyed when food is processed, cooked, or stored. Do not overcook vegetables. Steam vegetables with as little water as possible or microwave. Avoid boiling vegetables; the water will drain off many of the B vitamins. Much of this vitamin is lost when cereals are refined, thus the necessity of eating whole grains.

Optimal Supplementation: The RDA for this vitamin is probably sufficient. For healthy people, there is no evidence to show that more than the RDA is necessary for optimal health.

Toxicity: Megadoses of folate may cause convulsions in epileptics. Otherwise there are no reported incidences of problems with overdose. However, this drug is stored in the liver, which leads some nutrition experts to advise against taking large doses over an extended period of time.

If you suffer from pernicious anemia (a result of a vitamin B_{12} deficiency) taking large doses of folate may alleviate your obvious symptoms of anemia without curing the underlying condition. However, while taking folate and appearing to be healthy, victims of pernicious anemia may suffer neurological damage. It is recommended that folate supplementation be limited to not more than 400 micrograms a day. At that level, pernicious anemia symptoms will not be masked. Anyone suspected of suffering anemia of any kind should consult a physician.

Vitamin B_{12}

Chemical Name: Cobalamin

Main Functions in the Body:

• Metabolism of protein. The more protein you eat, the more vitamin B_{12} your body needs to process the protein.

• Needed for the creation of hemoglobin in red blood cells. (Interacts with folate.)

• Keeps the nervous system functioning correctly.

Vitamin B$_{12}$ Protects Against:

• Pernicious anemia: Your body cannot manufacture sufficient hemoglobin for your red blood cells without vitamin B$_{12}$. Victims of pernicious anemia may need intramuscular injections of vitamin B$_{12}$. Anyone suspected of suffering anemia of any kind should consult a physician.

• Megaloblastic anemia: Vitamin B$_{12}$, along with folate, is necessary for the proper formation of red blood cells. Megaloblastic anemia is characterized by malformed red blood cells.

• Sprue: This gastrointestinal disease causes diarrhea, intestinal lesions, and problems absorbing nutrients from the digestive tract. Vitamin B$_{12}$ activates folate to prevent this condition.

• Cancer: Vitamin B$_{12}$ may help the body fight off the effect of carcinogens, but this has not been conclusively established.

Signs of Deficiency: Overt deficiency causes pernicious anemia. Anyone suspected of suffering anemia of any kind should not attempt to treat it with vitamins but should consult a physician.

Vegetarians who consume no meat, eggs, or dairy foods may be at risk for deficiency because this vitamin is not found in vegetarian foods. Those who have had intestinal or gastric surgery are also at risk of deficiency. Symptoms of deficiency include sore tongue, numbness in extremities, weakness, and decreased sense of balance. The elderly may develop neuropsychiatric problems.

Recommended Dietary Allowance:

Adult men: 2 micrograms per day

Adult women: 2 micrograms per day

Number of Americans who get less than the RDA: 33 percent

Number of Americans who get less than 70 percent of the RDA: 15 percent

Best Food Sources: Milk, meat, eggs, cheese, kidney, liver. Not found in vegetarian foods.

Food Preparation Instructions: Avoid boiling foods and discarding the water. Boiling will drain off many B vitamins.

Optimal Supplementation: The RDA for this vitamin is sufficient for people in normal health. There is no evidence to show that more than the RDA is necessary for optimal health.

Toxicity: Megadoses of vitamin B_{12} have not been shown to cause problems at up to doses of 100 micrograms (50 times the RDA).

Biotin

Chemical Names of Related Compounds: Oxybiotin and biocytin

Main Functions in the Body:

- Necessary for the liberation of energy from carbohydrates
- Involved in the synthesis of fatty acids
- Necessary for the manufacture of some amino acids

Signs of Deficiency: Overt deficiency is rare. Usually, deficiency is only caused by eating a diet high in raw egg whites, which contain avidin, a chemical that prevents the absorption and use of biotin. Symptoms of deficiency include nausea and vomiting, depression, anorexia, pallor, hair loss, and dry, scaly skin.

Estimated Safe and Adequate Daily Range (there is no RDA for this vitamin):

Adult men: 30–100 micrograms per day

Adult women: 30–100 micrograms per day

Number of Americans who get less than the RDA: N/A

Number of Americans who get less than 70 percent of the RDA: N/A

Best Food Sources: Soy flour, corn, liver, egg yolk, yeast, and cereals

Food Preparation Instructions: Avoid eating raw egg whites, which contain avidin, a chemical that binds biotin and prevents the body from absorbing this vitamin.

Optimal Supplementation: There is no RDA for this vitamin, only a recommended range. Your intestinal bacteria can synthesize biotin, but it is not known if this source is available to the body.

Toxicity: Megadoses of biotin have never been reported to be harmful. Supplementation of up to 10 milligrams has been taken without ill effect.

Pantothenic Acid

Main Functions in the Body:

 • Necessary for the metabolism of carbohydrate, fat, and protein
 • Necessary for the manufacture of certain hormones and nervous system regulators

Signs of Deficiency: Overt deficiency is rare. Usually, deficiency is only caused by researchers who feed test subjects a special, limited diet. During World War II,

POWs suffered "burning feet" syndrome, which was blamed on pantothenic acid deficiency.

Estimated Safe and Adequate Daily Intake (there is no RDA for this vitamin):

Adult men: 4–7 milligrams per day

Adult women: 4–7 milligrams per day

Number of Americans who get less than the RDA: N/A

Number of Americans who get less than 70 percent of the RDA: N/A

Best Food Sources: Whole grains, legumes (peanuts, lentils, beans), meat

Food Preparation Instructions: Avoid overcooking foods.

Optimal Supplementation: There is no RDA for this vitamin, only a recommended range. Its wide availability in many foods probably makes it unnecessary to take this vitamin in supplement form.

Toxicity: Relatively nontoxic. Subjects in experiments have taken 10 grams a day without ill effect. Doses between 10 and 20 grams daily have caused water retention and diarrhea.

Minerals Most Frequently Taken As Supplements

Calcium

Chemical Names: Bones contain calcium phosphate

Main Functions in the Body:

- Used to form bones
- Necessary for conduction of nerve impulses

- Required for blood clots to form
- Calcium in cell membranes regulates fluid flow in and out of cells.
- Involved in the control of muscle contractions

Calcium Protects Against:

- Osteoporosis: Loss of calcium from the bones, most prevalent in postmenopausal women. Calcium by itself, however, does not prevent or cure osteoporosis. Some experts believe adequate calcium intake early in life, combined with exercise, can stave off this condition. Extra calcium ingested later in life may help reduce bone loss, but this assertion is contested by some experts.

Signs of Deficiency: Weakened bones.

Deficiency of calcium in children, teens, and young adults will often only make itself evident later in life, and then it is usually a problem for older women who suffer osteoporosis. As more men live longer, osteoporosis is expected also to become more of a problem among men.

Recommended Dietary Allowance:

Adult men: 1,200 milligrams per day until age 24, 800 milligrams per day for older men

Adult women: 1,200 milligrams per day until age 24, 800 milligrams per day for older women

Number of Americans who get less than the RDA: N/A

Number of Americans who get less than 70 percent of the RDA: N/A

Best Food Sources: Dairy products, small fish such as sardines eaten with bones, dark green leafy vegetables (broccoli, kale), tortillas made with lime

Food Preparation Instructions: No special care is necessary.

Optimal Supplementation: The RDA for this mineral is sufficient.

Toxicity: For adults, up to 2,500 milligrams a day has been reported safe, but in large amounts calcium causes constipation, urinary stones, and it may interfere with the absorption of iron and zinc and other minerals. Megadoses are not recommended.

Iron

Chemical Names: Stored in the body as ferritin and hemosiderin

Main Functions in the Body:

- Used to form hemoglobin in red blood cells
- Necessary for producing energy in the cells
- Necessary for formation of myoglobin in the muscles
- Necessary for proper function of the immune system

Iron Protects Against:

- Anemia
- Infectious diseases
- Impaired immune function

Sign of Deficiency: Anemia characterized by weakness, fatigue, pale skin, and lethargy. If you suspect you have anemia, see your doctor.

Deficiency of iron in children may cause short attention span, irritability, and problems in school. Children need the most iron as toddlers and then again in early adolescence.

Recommended Dietary Allowance:

Adult men: 10 milligrams

Adult women: 15 milligrams, during pregnancy 30 milligrams, while nursing 15 milligrams

Number of Americans who get less than the RDA: N/A

Number of Americans who get less than 70 percent of the RDA: N/A

Best Food Sources: Red meats, liver, dark green vegetables, legumes (beans, lentils), enriched grains, egg yolk

Food Preparation Instructions: No special care is necessary. Absorption from vegetable sources is enhanced by the simultaneous consumption of vitamin C. Adequate calcium also aids absorption.

Optimal Supplementation: Do not take more than the RDA for this mineral.

Toxicity: Highly dangerous. In children, death from iron overdose is the leading cause of poisoning from supplements. Keep all supplements that contain iron out of the reach of children. Never take large doses of iron; it can result in liver damage.

Zinc

Main Functions in the Body:

- Necessary for proper cell growth and repair
- Necessary for function of more than 100 enzymes
- Necessary for proper function of the immune system
- Aids in function of taste and smell

- Must be present for proper wound healing
- Zinc is present in high levels in many tissues including the prostate, pancreas, kidneys, and eyes.

Zinc Protects Against:

- Infectious diseases
- Impaired immune function
- Loss of ability to taste and smell odors

Signs of Deficiency: Skin rashes, slow growth, loss of appetite, reduced immune function, slow wound healing

In some countries of the Middle East, deficiency of zinc results in dwarfism.

Recommended Dietary Allowance:

Adult men: 15 milligrams

Adult women: 15 milligrams

Number of Americans who get less than the RDA: N/A

Number of Americans who get less than 70 percent of the RDA: N/A

Best Food Sources: Meat, cereals, liver, eggs, oysters and other seafood. The zinc found in grains is not readily absorbed.

Food Preparation Instructions: No special care is necessary.

Optimal Supplementation: Do not take more than the RDA for this mineral.

Toxicity: Amounts above the RDA can interfere with copper metabolism. Megadoses cause nausea and vomiting. High doses for a period of six weeks have caused impaired immune response and a decline in HDL cholesterol.

Chromium

Main Functions in the Body:

- Probably necessary for proper sugar metabolism
- May maintain healthy levels of HDL cholesterol

Chromium Possibly Protects Against:

- Heart disease (not conclusively established)
- Diabetes (not conclusively established)

Signs of Deficiency: Diabetes may be a result of chromium deficiency. Also, some cases of depressed HDL levels may be linked to a lack of this mineral.

Estimated Safe and Adequate Daily Dietary Intake:

Adult men: 50–100 micrograms

Adult women: 50–100 micrograms

Number of Americans who get less than the RDA: N/A

Number of Americans who get less than 70 percent of the RDA: N/A

Best Food Sources: Brewer's yeast, liver, American cheese, wheat germ

Food Preparation Instructions: No special care is necessary.

Optimal Supplementation: Do not take more than 200 micrograms of this mineral daily.

Toxicity: Little is known about chromium toxicity, but it is not thought to be dangerous. Megadoses are not recommended.

Selenium

Main Functions in the Body:

- Operates as part of enzymes that protect against oxidation caused by free radicals
- Interacts with vitamin E as an antioxidant

Selenium Protects Against:

- Keshan disease: A disease of the heart muscle

Signs of Deficiency: Difficult to discern. Population studies indicate that low levels of dietary selenium are associated with increased rates of cancer and heart disease.

Recommended Dietary Allowance:

Adult men: 70 micrograms

Adult women: 55 micrograms

Number of Americans who get less than the RDA: N/A

Number of Americans who get less than 70 percent of the RDA: N/A

Best Food Sources: Difficult to predict. Grains grown in soils containing high levels of selenium will be rich in this mineral. Liver, kidney, and seafood are generally good sources. Fruits and vegetables are usually poor sources.

Food Preparation Instructions: No special car is necessary.

Optimal Supplementation: Do not take more than 200 micrograms of this mineral daily.

Toxicity: Dangerous in large doses, can cause hair loss, deformed fingernails, diarrhea, and malaise

Magnesium

Main Functions in the Body:

- Necessary for proper formation of bones and teeth
- Takes part in many metabolic processes as constituent of more than 300 enzymes
- Necessary for muscle function
- Takes part in the release of energy from glycogen, or stored carbohydrates
- Necessary for transmission of nerve impulses

Magnesium Protects Against:

- Muscle weakness

Signs of Deficiency: Overt deficiency is rare. Deficiency may be characterized by nausea, irritability, heart abnormalities, mental confusion, and muscle spasms.

Recommended Dietary Allowance:

Adult men: 350 milligrams

Adult women: 280–300 milligrams

Number of Americans who get less than the RDA: N/A

Number of Americans who get less than 70 percent of the RDA: N/A

Best Food Sources: Unprocessed foods including whole grains, legumes (lentils, beans), and nuts. Bananas are the only fruit that is a good source of magnesium.

Food Preparation Instructions: No special care is necessary.

Optimal Supplementation: Do not take more than the RDA of this mineral.

Toxicity: Highly safe except for people with kidney disease. Normally, magnesium-containing drugs are the only causes of magnesium overdose.

12

Special Circumstances Requiring Supplementation

Note: Mention of a multivitamin supplement in these entries refers to a supplement containing the RDA for all of the water- and fat-soluble vitamins.

If You Exercise

If you maintain your physical fitness by exercising—working out with weights, swimming, running, bicycling, or other strenuous activities—you may need extra doses of antioxidant vitamins (vitamins C and E and beta-carotene) as well as riboflavin.

Studies show that exercise, while it conditions the cardiovascular system, results in added oxidative stress in muscles and other tissues. Antioxidant supplements can help repair this damage.

Riboflavin, which is needed for carbohydrate metabolism, is also an important nutrient for exercisers. If you rarely consume dairy products, which are a main source of this nutrient, you should consider a supplement containing the RDA for riboflavin.

If You Are Over Forty Years Old

As we age, our absorption of nutrients from our food may become less efficient and our bodies may be less able to store vitamins. Added to that problem, we often eat less as our metabolism slows, and we sometimes fall into poor eating habits. Some experts point out that older citizens frequently show signs of deficiency in the B vitamins as well as vitamin C.

This group should consider a multivitamin plus extra C and possibly a B supplement.

If You Use Alcohol

Heavy drinking is responsible for B vitamin deficiencies as well as many other health problems. While extra supplements of the B vitamins may help drinkers, it is better to drink in moderation or not at all to restore an adequate vitamin status.

Heavy drinkers should probably stay away from taking beta-carotene supplements, since studies indicate this nutrient may cause liver damage when accompanied by large amounts of alcohol.

If You Smoke

Cigarette smoke, like other air pollutants, destroys the vitamins in your body, particularly the antioxidant vitamins. All smokers should take a multivitamin plus extra helpings of vitamins C and E and beta-carotene. They should also eat a diet high in leafy green vegetables, since studies show these have been associated with lower levels of cancer.

To acquire optimal vitamin status, cigarette smokers should stop smoking.

If You Are a Woman Who Uses Contraceptives

The use of oral contraceptives can lower the levels of vitamins circulating in your body. In particular, you will need extra amounts of vitamin C, vitamin B_6, and niacin. Therefore, pay special attention to eating a diet containing many leafy green vegetables and legumes. Supplementation with a multivitamin is also a good idea, as is taking a supplement containing some extra vitamin C.

Men and Women of Childbearing Years

Any woman who is pregnant should consult a physician and take the multivitamin that the doctor prescribes. Recent studies affirm the importance of pregnant women taking a supplement containing folic acid to lower the chance of their babies being born with birth defects (most importantly, neural tube defects, see page 73). Pregnant women also should not take megadoses of vitamins because these vitamins can affect the fetus.

Men who want to be fathers should take vitamin C. Seminal fluid contains high concentrations of this vitamin and some experts believe that vitamin C is essential for sperm health.

Women who breast-feed should also take multivitamin supplements. They should consult a physician or registered dietitian for dietary information.

Dieters

Anyone on a restricted or special diet should, at minimum, take a multivitamin supplement. Even the most reactionary of dietitians and doctors now recognize that those who restrict their calorie intake or follow other restrictive dietary guidelines usually will not consume the RDA for all of the vitamins.

Caution: You should not go on a very restricted diet without consulting a knowledgeable physician or a registered dietitian.

Coffee, Tea, and Cola Drinkers

If you consume drinks containing large amounts of caffeine (this includes other soft drinks besides cola), this drug may be removing vitamins from your body, especially the water-soluble vitamins. The tannins in tea may also restrict vitamin absorption. Use a multivitamin.

Very High Fiber Diets

Eating a diet high in fiber has many health benefits, but fibrous meals may possibly limit your absorption of vitamins. Try taking a multivitamin with your least fibrous meal of the day.

13

Questions and Answers
About Vitamins

Q: I've been told that taking large amounts of vitamin C can produce kidney stones. Is this a real danger?

A: While the supposed risk of developing kidney stones from taking large doses of vitamin C has been promulgated by many different sources, the actual chances of this happening are very, very remote. As a matter of fact, it has never been reliably shown that taking vitamin C has ever given anybody kidney stones.

How did this kidney stone myth start? One of the ways in which ascorbic acid (vitamin C) is processed in the body results in the formation of oxalic acid, a chemical that is sometimes a factor in the formation of kidney stones. That has led some scientists to hypothesize that large doses of vitamin C could produce enough oxalic acid to yield kidney stones.

However, when researchers looked at how much oxalic acid people actually produce when given vitamin C, the results have not been consistent. In one study, about 5 percent of vitamin C takers were producing increased amounts of oxalic acid after taking up to 9 grams daily of the nutrient. Another study found no increase in oxalic acid after volunteers took more than 3 grams a day for up to six months.

In any case, there are only three reports of people who had kidney stones and also took vitamin C, and there was no evidence that it was the vitamin C that gave them the kidney stones. It might have been coincidental.

Many researchers who have given people large doses of vitamin C believe the stuff is practically nontoxic at almost any dosage. Certainly, in many large-scale experiments where cancer patients took up to 10 grams of the vitamin for up to two years, nobody reported getting kidney stones, so the danger of this happening is somewhere between nonexistent and remote.

Incidentally, until recently, doctors recommended that people with a tendency to develop stones should cut back on their calcium intake on the theory that stones are made of calcium, therefore calcium-rich foods may stimulate stone formation. Recent studies have shown that this recommendation is not only incorrect but the exact opposite of what is true: Those who eat the least amount of calcium develop more stones than other people. The new recommendation is to eat more calcium and also consume fruits and vegetables that contain other minerals that may help keep kidney stones from forming. This is just another example of how the science of nutrition and vitamins is still evolving.

Q: When I take 4 grams of vitamin C a day, I get stomach pains and diarrhea. What should I do?

A: You probably should take less of the vitamin. While large doses of this vitamin probably can't really hurt you, it does have an effect on the bowels (as you've discovered). The dosage at which this happens varies from individual to individual. Some people also experience flatulence, nausea, and, supposedly, vomiting at high doses. None of the studies in which this occurred, according to Dr. Gladys Block of the National Cancer Institute and Dr. Marilyn Menkes of the Johns Hopkins School of Hygiene and Public Health, included groups taking placebos, so it is not certain that these reactions were to vitamin C. The nausea might have been produced by a psychological reaction to taking pills rather than from the vitamin itself.

On the other hand, many individuals do not seem to be bothered by any stomach problems at any dose of vitamin C. It is possible, according to Drs. Block and Menkes, that cancer patients or anybody else undergoing severe biological stress may be more tolerant of large doses of vitamin C than people who are healthy.

Some experts even suggest that how well your bowels react may be an indicator of how much vitamin C you need. In other words, if it doesn't give you diarrhea at high doses, then maybe you need high doses. But that, of course, is just a hypothesis. To figure out how much vitamin C you can tolerate and not be uncomfortable, gradually cut down on your daily dosage until the diarrhea stops.

Don't cut back on your vitamin C intake too quickly. Some experts believe that suddenly not taking vitamin C after taking large doses for a long time may give you a kind of "rebound scurvy," a short-term shortage of vitamin C that occurs because your body has become accustomed to such high doses. Although this has never been firmly established, it's advisable to decrease dosages gradually.

If you are pregnant and taking vitamins, it is also a good idea to moderate your vitamin C intake. There are a few cases on record of infants suffering scurvy because they were born to mothers taking large doses of vitamin C, so go easy while you are pregnant and discuss this situation with your obstetrician and pediatrician.

Q: Doesn't taking vitamin C destroy the vitamin B$_{12}$ in your body?

A: This is another myth that started in the laboratory but seems to have no truth to it when applied to the real world.

In the 1970s, scientists experimenting with foods found evidence, they thought, that showed that when up to half a gram of vitamin C was present in a meal, it destroyed any vitamin B$_{12}$ that was contained in the foods. Other scientists doing the same experiment a slightly different way found that it wasn't so.

In follow-up studies, in real people, it has been shown that people taking 3 or 4 grams of vitamin C per day did not experience any loss of vitamin B$_{12}$.

Q: I'm supposed to take a test for blood in my feces (occult blood), and my doctor told me that the vitamin C I take will interfere with the test. What should I do?

A: Follow your doctor's instructions and stop taking vitamin C two or three days before you have the test. If you have a lot of vitamin C in your system, it could produce a false positive on this test.

As for other tests such as colorimetric tests for uric acid, glucose, bilirubin, SGOT, SGPT, and LDH, vitamin C will not produce any tangible interference with your results.

However, before taking any medical tests or medications, discuss your diet and vitamin supplementation with your doctor to make sure that your vitamins will not interfere with whatever your doctor has planned. For instance, vitamin C has been shown to alter the action of blood thinners (warfarin and other anticoagulants), so if you are taking this type of medication, it is not a good idea to take big doses of vitamin C. In any case, you should discuss this with your doctor.

Q: Can vitamin C affect how much iron you absorb from foods?

A: When you consume vitamin C along with your meals, this nutrient will increase the amount of iron you absorb from vegetarian foods (to experts these foods are known as nonheme sources of iron). The vitamin C you take will not affect how much iron your body will take in from meats (heme sources). Normally, the iron you take in from meat is better absorbed than the iron in vegetables because of an iron-absorption factor in meat that scientists have still not been able to isolate. (Nutrition is, after all, still a young science.)

The fact that vitamin C increases iron absorption should not be a problem for most people and may be a benefit for some. If you are a woman eating a vegetarian diet who is afraid she is not getting enough iron, vitamin C acts as an aid to absorbing more of this mineral.

On the other hand, there are some relatively rare instances when people may not want to be exposed to too much iron. People suffering from a condition called hemochromatosis, a genetic problem that affects an individual's iron absorption, and people with beta-thalassemia who receive regular blood transfusions should usually avoid taking large doses of vitamin C. In these cases and anytime you have a medical problem that may be influenced by your vitamin intake, you should consult with your doctor and follow her/his advice.

Q: I've been thinking of taking tryptophan supplements. I have been told that tryptophan can help you sleep and your body uses it to make niacin. I can't find this supplement in the stores. Can I order it in the mail? How much should I take?

A: Don't take any. While it is true that your body uses the amino acid tryptophan to make niacin, taking tryptophan supplements is a very poor way to get this nutrient. People have become very sick and died from taking tryptophan supplements, and no one knows why.

Tryptophan would appear to be a benign substance. It is an amino acid contained in milk, and chances are you eat plenty of this substance in your food already. A few years ago, while tryptophan supplements were enjoying increased popularity (supposedly the supplements could help you sleep, they alleviated some symptoms of premenstrual syndrome, and helped some people overcome bulimia), people began to suffer eosinophilia-myalagia syndrome, a severe problem with some of their blood cells.

Because of deaths associated with tryptophan, the Food and Drug Administration has forbidden the sale of tryptophan supplements in the United States. It is possible that the people who died from taking tryptophan actually were killed by contaminants in the supplements, which were mainly made in Japan by a process that used bacteria. To this day, no one knows what caused the problem, so don't buy or take this supplement. If you have old tryptophan supplements in the house, throw them out or flush them down the toilet.

Q: I'm not an alcoholic, but I enjoy wine or beer every night with dinner. Can taking vitamins offset the bad effects of alcohol?

A: Probably not, although many people who drink too much may suffer from several different vitamin deficiencies. Certainly you should be taking a multivitamin, but the most important thing you should do, for health reasons, is to make sure you drink in moderation.

In some cases, mixing large doses of vitamins and alcohol may be hazardous to your health. One study, done with animals, has shown that taking substantial amounts of beta-carotene while imbibing significant amounts of alcohol may harm your liver, the organ that has to process both of these chemicals when it enters your body.

An important rule to remember is that vitamins can help a healthy lifestyle be healthier, but they can't be relied on to offset poor habits like drinking and smoking.

Q: What's the best way to cook vegetables so that their vitamins aren't destroyed?

A: Microwave them in little or no water. If you cook them on the stove top, steam them rather than boiling them. Always use as little water as possible. Water will remove many of the vitamins and minerals from foods. Many of the B vitamins are especially susceptible to being leached out by water.

When cooking fresh vegetables, don't prepare them ahead of time. Always cook them just before eating. If you can avoid it, don't dice them into small pieces. Vitamin C is destroyed by light and air, so the more surface area that is exposed, the less of this vitamin will still be in the food when you consume it.

Don't be afraid to eat frozen vegetables. Because of improvements in the way produce is frozen, most of the vitamins are retained in frozen foods. As a matter of fact, some studies have shown that if your supermarket lets its produce sit on the shelves for very long, the frozen vegetables may actually retain more of their vitamins than the fresh offerings.

Q: Does frozen orange juice have any vitamin C left in it?

A: Almost as much as fresh juice (about 20 percent less). The way concentrate is made and frozen today retains most of the vitamin C. As long as it is stored at 0° F. in your freezer, most of that vitamin C should still be there. The juices available in cartons in the refrigerated section of the supermarket should have about the same amount of vitamin C (about 100 milligrams per cup).

After you mix the concentrate with water or open a carton, the juice should be consumed as soon as possible, since vitamin C is destroyed by light and air. If you keep the reconstituted juice around for more than three days, it will suffer a substantial loss in vitamin C, depending on the temperature in your refrigerator and how much light it is exposed to.

Q: A friend of mine eats carrots every day. The palms of his hands have turned yellowish. Is this a dangerous condition?

A: Aside from the fact that you may begin to look like a giant carrot, the yellow-orange tinge in the skin that appears from taking in too much beta-carotene and the other carotenoids is probably harmless, according to experts. These substances are the pigments that give carrots and some other fruits and vegetables their characteristic color. If you eat a pound or more of carrots a day, or consume other carotene-rich fruits and vegetables, these colorings will find a new home in your fatty tissue just below your skin. Since much of this fatty tissue is in the palms of your hands and the soles of your feet, these will tend to turn the most yellow.

Apparently, you can get seriously hooked on these veggies. There have been reports of people addicted to carrots who had difficulty cutting them out of their diet. In Europe, Czech psychiatrists reported that three people who ate up to ten large carrots a day suffered withdrawal symptoms when a carrot shortage forced them to stop eating so many carrots. American doctors think the addiction was more psychological than physical and was related to eating disorders and other mental problems.

If your friend is tired of being called yellow and does not have a psychological addiction to carrots, all she or he has to do is cut back on the carrots for a while and the yellow-orange color will slowly dissipate. Remind your friend not to indulge in too much alcohol while eating a heavy diet of beta-carotene. That can be hard on your liver.

Q: Is it better to take natural vitamins?

A: This is one of those questions that probably can't be satisfactorily answered. First of all, the majority of chemists will tell you that there is no chemical difference between a natural vitamin and an artificial one. According to this view, the chemical structure is the same and your body can't tell them apart. The one exception is vitamin E, which some experts say is better used by the body in its natural form, d-alpha-tocopherol. Other than that, no matter which form of vitamin you swallow, it will have the same effect in your body.

Of course, purists insist on natural vitamins, although their belief in the natural form may be based more on wishful thinking than on scientific evidence. In any case, with the exception noted above, no one has ever performed a reliable study to tell if there is a difference in health effects between vitamins extracted from natural sources and vitamins cooked up from scratch in the lab.

Also at issue is the definition of natural. There really isn't a good one. Even when vitamins are extracted from food, the extraction process is so complex and drawn out that there hardly seems to be anything natural about the end result. The extraction process often involves the application of many different chemicals, so the vitamin that comes out can hardly be said to be unprocessed.

The only really natural vitamins are those that are to be found in food. You could say that food is a vitamin's natural habitat. There it is accompanied by other nutrients and may be present in many different forms. For instance, while you can take beta-carotene in a pill, when you eat it in a carrot or other vegetable, it is accompanied by other types of carotenes, fiber, vitamin C, and many other nutrients. There are many factors in food that are vital to our health that we haven't isolated and synthesized.

Similarly, when you take vitamin E capsules—even in a natural formulation—you usually are swallowing alpha-tocopherol, only one form of the vitamin. Some vitamin pills do contain several tocopherols (see below), but they probably won't be present in the same ratio as they would be in food. Does this make a difference to your health? Probably not. Is this an argument not to take vitamins? No. But it does mean you shouldn't be too hung up on taking natural vitamins, and you should eat a healthful diet that contains plenty of fruits and vegetables that contain many nutrients most of us get too little of.

Q: My vitamin E bottle says it contains dl-alpha-tocopherol. What does that mean?

A: Vitamin E is available in two forms: dl-alpha-tocopherol and d-alpha-tocopherol. The so-called natural form is d-alpha, while the synthetic form of the vitamin is dl-alpha. These are traditional terms of long standing and most vitamin manufacturers still use them. More recently, an international agreement stipulated that natural vitamin E would now be known as RRR-alpha-tocopherol, while the synthetic vitamin E is to be called all-rac-alpha-tocopherol.

When it comes to measuring out the vitamin E for your vitamin E capsules, the basic measurement has usually been the international unit. This unit is a measure of how much use your body should get from the vitamin (also known as its biological activity). According to the committee that draws up the RDAs, an international unit of vitamin E is defined as the amount of vitamin E that provides the usefulness of 1 milligram of the synthetic tocopherol (the dl-alpha form). Because the synthetic vitamin E is only 74 percent as active as the natural form, it takes less of the natural E to give you the same effect as the synthetic form. According to the chemists, however, vitamin E capsules marked with an equal amount of international units, whether synthetic or natural, will be utilized equally in the human body.

Q: I heard that smoking uses up the vitamins in your body. Is this true?

A: Yes. Smoking does destroy a significant portion of the antioxidants circulating in your blood and in your internal organs. Consequently, many nutrition experts recommend that smokers take extra amounts of vitamin C, beta-carotene, and vitamin E.

That doesn't mean you can safely smoke and depend on supplements of antioxidant vitamins to protect your health. Your best bet is to give up the use of all tobacco products if you wish to live to enjoy a ripe old age. Every year more than 100,000 Americans die of lung cancer, and most of these cases are linked to smoking. (This represents more than 2,000 people daily, every day of the year.) Smoking has also been linked to cancer of the mouth, the larynx, the esophagus, the bladder, even cancer of the tongue. This nasty habit also causes heart disease.

Consequently, the most reliable course of action is to give up smoking, eat a reasonable diet, and take vitamins. Studies show that the sooner you give up smoking the better. Ex-smokers still have a slightly higher risk of disease than those who never smoked, but the younger you are when you quit the habit, the lower your chances are of suffering a smoking-related illness.

Q: I've heard that taking extra vitamin D will make my bones stronger. How does this work?

A: While vitamin D does play a role in regulating the formation of the bone, for most people, taking supplements of this vitamin is not a good idea. Taking excessive amounts of vitamin D is potentially poisonous, especially for children. Too much of this nutrient can cause permanent damage to the kidneys and the cardiovascular system.

Vitamin D is added to milk and your skin can make this vitamin, so taking supplements is almost always unnecessary. However, if you hardly ever get any sun (for instance, if you must avoid the sunshine because of a medical condition) and you never drink milk, you may need small supplements of vitamin D. In that case, you should consult a knowledgeable doctor about the possible benefits of supplementation. Don't decide to take this vitamin on your own to solve what could be a serious medical problem. Chances are, a few minutes in the sun every week will supply you with enough of this vitamin.

If you are worried about your bone strength but do not suffer from osteoporosis or osteomalacia, a better idea than taking vitamin D is to perform ample amounts of weight-bearing exercise (such as walking, running, and weight lifting) and eat plenty of calcium-rich foods such as dairy products and leafy green vegetables.

Q: Are chelated vitamins better for you?

A: While some minerals are absorbed better by the body when they are chelated, vitamins are absorbed very well without this process. Chelation refers to the combining of minerals with metallic ions that increase their efficient absorption from the intestinal tract.

What that means is that the form of the mineral is changed to better enable the body to break it apart so that it can be taken in more thoroughly through the walls of the intestine. (In Greek *chela* means claw, referring to the fact that the chelating agent forms a bond with the mineral in a claw-shaped structure.)

Vitamins do not need to be chelated to be efficiently absorbed and used by the body.

Q: Is it true that lettuce has no vitamins?

A: Iceberg lettuce, the most popular lettuce in the United States, has very few vitamins, but other kinds of lettuce are rich in nutrients. For instance, romaine, a leafy green lettuce, has fair amounts of beta-carotene, vitamin C, fiber, and minerals.

As a general rule, the darker the lettuce, the more vitamins (beta-carotene and other carotenes give the lettuce its color). Iceberg lettuce is practically devoid of vitamins or fiber, although it is crunchy and people like its taste.

Q: Can you become addicted to vitamins?

A: Not in the sense that you can become addicted to drugs, but some experts suggest that if you take large amounts of vitamin C daily and then suddenly stop cold turkey, you may experience rebound scurvy, a type of vitamin C deficiency resulting from your body's being accustomed to megadoses of vitamin C (see page 221).

Q: Is it safe to take dolomite or bone meal in order to make sure you are getting enough calcium?

A: While both of these types of supplements supply adequate and absorbable forms of calcium, they also have been found to be contaminated with significant levels of lead and other metals including mercury and arsenic that are dangerous to your health. It is not recommended that you take these types of supplements. Better to get your calcium from nonfat dairy foods or other types of calcium supplements.

Q: Do I need to keep my vitamin bottles in a special place?

A: Vitamins in capsule and pill form are generally very stable, but to make sure that they remain at full potency, they should be stored in a cool, dark place. The refrigerator is not recommended because of the possibility of the buildup of moisture in the bottles that could degrade the supplements.

Wherever you choose to store them, be sure that they are inaccessible to children who can poison themselves with these pills. This is especially important if you keep supplements containing iron in the house. In large doses, iron is very toxic. When children ingest large doses, it destroys their livers. Iron supplements represent the leading cause of fatal poisonings from supplements among young children every year.

Q: My friend takes comfrey pepsin capsules. What are their benefits?

A: While no benefits have been scientifically proven for these types of supplements, there have been reports of risk involved with this type of capsule. One woman developed serious illness after taking these capsules for about four months. An analysis of these capsules revealed the presence of types of chemicals called alkaloids that potentially could cause liver damage or cancer, so it is best to avoid these capsules.

Q: Do fiber supplements benefit your health or help you lose weight?

A: There is little evidence to support either of those claims. Experts believe that the studies done to show that fiber supplements helped people lose weight were not designed properly and really didn't prove their usefulness for weight loss.

Dietary fiber is a complex group of substances that includes all of the parts of plants that your body is unable to digest. As these substances pass through your body, they engender many chemical reactions that benefit your health. They speed elimination of stools and help prevent constipation and diverticulitis. Some forms of fiber can lower cholesterol, others are associated with a reduced risk of colon cancer. To make sure you are getting an adequate supply of a wide range of fibers, it is best to eat a diet filled with as many fruits, vegetables, whole grains, and legumes (beans, lentils, etc.) as possible.

Each one of the fibers in vegetarian foods seems to play a slightly different, beneficial role in your body.

Scientists have not yet been able to identify all of these fibers or their functions, so it's a sure bet that there are fibers in food that have not been isolated and put into fiber pills—a good reason to rely on food rather than supplements for your fiber. Also, fiber is a bulky substance that doesn't lend itself to concentration in pill form. For all those reasons, it is better to rely on foods than pills to get enough of this nutrient.

Q: Is it better to take your daily vitamins all at once or spread them out over the whole day?

A: Depending on how many supplements you are taking, it's a good idea to spread out your vitamin intake over the course of the day, a little with each meal, although taking a multivitamin just once during the day is acceptable. If you take one single large dose in the morning, for example, chances are more of the vitamins will pass through you without being absorbed. A little at a time gives your digestive system more of a chance to take in proportionately more of the vitamins you swallow.

Don't take your vitamins on an empty stomach. Taking them with food will help your body take in the vitamins and use them efficiently, since there are many cofactors in food that enhance vitamin absorption.

If you take vitamin E and/or beta-carotene, make sure you take these nutrients with a meal that contains some fat. The absorption of these fat-soluble vitamins is aided by the presence of fatty acids in the digestive tract.

You should also be sure to take your vitamins with water or juice. Don't swallow them dry, since water will also help in your body's utilization of nutrients.

Q: Why are some products fortified with vitamins while others are enriched? How come white bread

is enriched while whole wheat bread doesn't have vitamins added?

A: Food products such as white bread and white flour are said to be enriched when the food manufacturer puts back some of the nutrients that have been taken out during the refinement process. All wheat flour starts out as whole wheat. When it is made into white flour (and subsequently white bread), it loses almost all of its fiber, as well as the vitamins folic acid, vitamin B_6, thiamine, riboflavin, and niacin, and the minerals zinc, chromium, magnesium, and iron. Enrichment gives it back its iron, thiamine, riboflavin, and niacin. If you want those other healthy nutrients, you have to eat whole wheat bread.

Fortified foods have had nutrients added that would not usually be present in significant amounts. For instance, milk is fortified with the vitamins A and D, two nutrients that are not naturally present in such quantities. Other dairy foods, such as yogurt and ice cream are not usually fortified and do not contain very much of these vitamins.

Many breakfast cereals are fortified with a wide variety of vitamins and minerals that they would not normally contain. While these cereals add to your vitamin intake, in many cases it is not certain that all of these vitamins are present in forms your body can absorb efficiently.

Q: Is it worthwhile to have your hair analyzed to assess your vitamin status?

A: While analyzing hair has been used in studies to tell whether or not groups of people have been exposed to dangerous heavy metals such as lead or mercury, nutrition experts discount its usefulness for figuring out vitamin deficiencies. A big problem with hair analysis is the lack of generally accepted standards for interpreting what the lab finds in your hair. No one has ever figured out how the vitamin level in your hair correlates with the vitamin levels in your blood or other parts of your body.

Since there are no laboratory standards for hair analysis, experts feel that commercial labs frequently overstate their results in order to sell more supplements meant to overcome deficiencies that are supposedly found. One researcher reported that when he sent hair samples from the same two people to thirteen different labs, he got back thirteen different results. The labs also could not agree on what a normal result should have been. About half of the responding labs recommended various amounts of supplements to alleviate the so-called deficiencies.

If you are really worried about your vitamin status, find a doctor who will prescribe a blood analysis. That kind of test will be much more accurate than a test of your hair.

Q: Sometimes, after I take a B vitamin complex, my urine looks bright yellow. Is this dangerous? Why does this happen?

A: No, it's perfectly safe. What is happening is that your body is eliminating excess riboflavin, which gives urine a yellow or yellowish green appearance. There is no evidence that it can hurt you. As you can see, the body easily eliminates any riboflavin that it does not need.

Is that excess riboflavin doing you any good if you are just losing it soon after taking your vitamin? The answer depends on who you ask. Many nutrition experts will tell you that you are wasting your money on your B supplements because all you are accomplishing is the creation of expensive urine. Other experts argue that having these vitamins pass through the urinary tract may help the health of that part of the body.

In any case, you probably don't need to take the B vitamins in amounts much larger than the RDA, and the real test for how useful they are for your health is how you feel. If they are part of your supplement program and they help you feel in optimal health, then there is no reason to stop taking them.

Q: I have heard that if I take my vitamins with a meal that contains high-fiber foods, the fiber will keep my body from absorbing the vitamins. Is that true?

A: A few years ago, there was some concern that eating a high-fiber diet would interfere with mineral absorption. Many high-fiber foods and bran contain a substance called phytic acid or phytate, which can theoretically tie up zinc and other nutrients and prevent your body from taking them in.

Most experts doubt that high-fiber foods or the phytate they contain will significantly compromise your nutrient intake. However, it is probably not a good idea to take all of your vitamins with extremely high-fiber meals or at the same time as taking bran or eating cereal that has had bran added to it. As I've said earlier, take your vitamins over the course of the day to enhance absorption.

Don't overdo the bran, either. Some nutrition researchers worry that taking large doses of bran over a long period of time could have unforeseen effects that no one has yet observed. It is better to eat a wide variety of fibrous foods instead of overdosing on one type.

Q: Can you get all the vitamins you need on a vegetarian diet?

A: Except for vitamin B_{12}, even strict vegetarians can get all the nutrients they need from a vegetarian diet without eating any meat. If a vegetarian eats foods such as cheese, eggs, and milk, even this vitamin will be present in the diet. Vitamin D may also be a concern for strict vegetarians who eschew dairy products, since this nutrient is primarily available in fortified milk.

As a general rule, vegetarians and anyone following any kind of restricted diet should take a multivitamin. Vegetarians should also be sure to eat plenty of dark green vegetables, which have ample amounts of calcium and, if they are concerned about iron absorption, they should have a vitamin C supplement or eat food rich in vitamin C, such as citrus fruit and kiwi fruit, with each meal to enhance iron absorption. Without vitamin C, iron in vegetarian foods is not absorbed efficiently.

Except for these few concerns, vegetarians often consume more of the vitamins C, E, and beta-carotene than people who eat meals heavy with meat. Many studies show that vegetarians weigh less, have a lower risk of heart disease and certain forms of cancer, and enjoy other health benefits as well.

Q: Are there any vitamins that can relieve premenstrual syndrome (PMS)?

A: Many substances have been touted as cures or alleviators of PMS, but none have been proven to be effective for large groups of women. While vitamin E, vitamin A, and magnesium have been advertised in over-the-counter preparations for PMS, the most popular has been vitamin B_6.

Some women swear by the effectiveness of B_6, but there is little scientific evidence showing that it works to relieve PMS. One factor that confounds scientists is that in double-blind studies, where half the female subjects were given placebos and half were given B_6, the placebo group often showed as much relief as the B_6 group.

According to some experts, vitamin B_6 should be used with caution because amounts as low as 500 milligrams a day have produced adverse effects such as numbness in the extremities, trouble using the muscles, as well as burning and pins-and-needles feelings in the skin. The RDA for vitamin B_6 for adult women is 5 milligrams a day, and it should not be taken in doses much larger than that amount.

Q: Does bee pollen contain vitamins that can increase stamina?

A: Even though bee pollen has been sold as an endurance builder for long-distance runners and others, there is no evidence that it helps you run faster or improves your health or athletic performance in any way. There is also some reason to believe that some products marketed as bee pollen are bogus and have never been touched by bees.

In addition to its worthlessness as a performance booster, bee pollen may cause allergic reactions in some people. This material also contains a relatively high concentration of nucleic acids that may cause problems in people at risk for kidney disease or gout.

Stay off the bee pollen. Aside from bringing in revenue for bee pollen packagers, a jar of bee pollen won't help you and may just be a jar full of trouble.

Q: I sometimes take mineral oil as a laxative, but now I've been warned it can take vitamins out of your body. Is it safe to use?

A: Ingesting mineral oil for any reason is ill advised. Your body cannot digest this substance and it may very well react with other nutrients you have consumed.

As an indigestible fat, mineral oil in your digestive

tract picks up fat-soluble vitamins and eliminates them before you can absorb them. It is a particularly effective solvent for beta-carotenes and the other carotenes, so taking mineral oil will in effect rob your body of some important antioxidants that are vital to your health. That is why using mineral oil on salad as some diets advise is an especially bad idea. The carotenes from the green and yellow vegetables will pass right through you uselessly.

If you want to avoid too much fat in your salad dressing, buy a ready-made low-fat dressing or use nonfat yogurt. Instead of using mineral oil as a laxative, try eating a diet high in fiber, which relieves constipation in many people. A regular program of exercise also helps.

Q: I've heard that there are vitamins in cabbage that can prevent cancer. What are they?

A: Cabbage is a member of the family of foods known as the cruciferous vegetables and there is evidence that chemicals in these foods can help prevent cancer. The protective factors in this group of vegetables are not vitamins, they are substances called indoles, which have been found in the lab to inhibit cancer growth and slow the interactions in the body that can give rise to carcinogenic chemicals.

The cruciferous vegetables include kale, cauliflower, and broccoli as well as cabbage. These vegetables also usually include a good supply of vitamins, minerals, and fiber as well as indoles, and they should be an important part of your diet.

Q: A friend of mine puts sodium bicarbonate in the water when cooking vegetables to make them look greener. Does this affect the food's vitamins?

A: Yes, and you should never use it. Sometimes vegetables, because of aging, loose their luster and their green color grows dull. Sodium bicarbonate prevents the chlorophyll in the vegetables from undergoing the chemical changes that produce this dull green, but it destroys thiamine and vitamin C. If your vegetables are too old to look attractive, throw them out and cook fresher ones. They'll look and taste better and your body will derive more nutrients from them.

Q: For years I've taken niacin to control my blood cholesterol. The niacin I used to take made me feel uncomfortable. I felt tingling and a flushing sensation in my face. Now I've switched to a time-release capsule that doesn't make me uncomfortable. Is a time-release capsule a good way to take niacin?

A: First of all, anyone who takes megadoses of niacin to control cholesterol should be under a doctor's supervision. Over a long period of time, taking large amounts of this vitamin can cause serious medical problems such as liver damage. Your physician should periodically give you blood tests to make sure this isn't happening to you.

Feeling uncomfortably warm and getting a tingling and flushing feeling in parts of your body, particularly your face, is a common side effect to taking niacin. It is not unusual. Some people hate these sensations while other people do not seem to mind. Even though you may be grateful that your new niacin pills are not causing you any discomfort, the fact is, they also may not be allowing your body to absorb much niacin. Without those symptoms, you cannot be sure that any of the niacin is actually entering your body.

In the past, laboratory tests of several time-release niacin formulas showed that some of them, when subjected to conditions similar to those in your digestive tract, were not even halfway dissolved after twelve hours.

A better way to take your niacin and avoid the strong side effects that come on after a single megadose is to take several small doses during the day. Try taking your supplements after eating so the food in your stomach can slow down your niacin absorption. As time-release formulations travel through your body, they may never release enough niacin until it is too late to be absorbed.

Q: I try to buy foods that have the highest vitamin content listed on the labels, but how accurate are these labels?

A: Not very. Food and Drug Administration (FDA) standards require that food labels have a 20 percent accuracy. That means that the nutrients in the food inside the package can contain 20 percent more or 20 percent less than what is indicated on the label. If a container of juice indicates that a serving contains 60 milligrams of vitamin C, for instance, it may actually contain anywhere from 48 milligrams to 72 milligrams.

The rationale behind this allowance for error is that food varies in its nutrient content from batch to batch. Not every can of orange juice concentrate will contain the same amounts of vitamin C and other nutrients, so the FDA reasons that not every glass of orange juice can be expected to conform to an exact amount of nutrients. It's unrealistic to expect that kind of accuracy.

But if you are dieting and counting calories and nutrients, this inaccuracy in labels is disconcerting. A helping of soup that is labeled as 100 calories may actually contain up to 120, or it could be as low as 80.

When it comes to supplements, the FDA supposedly requires that all vitamin pills and capsules contain at least the amount listed on the label, but, in fact, the FDA does not presently have the money or personpower to put any teeth into these requirements. Don't put too much stock into the expiration dates on vitamin labels, either. Each company invents its own based on arbitrary standards that do not require substantiation from either the FDA nor the United States Pharmacopeia, the organization that sets drug standards.

Q: How many calories are in vitamins?

A: Since vitamins are used as coenzymes in the body—they join with enzymes to speed chemical and metabolic reactions—these nutrients essentially have no calories. Some vitamin preparations contain minimal amounts of starch and sugar, which are believed to help your body absorb vitamins more efficiently. The small amounts of sugar or starch in your vitamin pills make no appreciable contribution to your daily calorie intake.

Q: First I heard that vitamin C keeps you from getting colds, then I heard that it doesn't work against colds, and now somebody else has told me that it shortens your colds. Who is right?

A: Years ago, vitamin C advocates proclaimed this vitamin as the silver bullet in the war against the common cold. But their arguments were overstated. When researchers ran large-scale studies testing vitamin C's ability to prevent the common cold, they were partially disappointed. In the tests, even people who took large amounts of vitamin C caught just as many colds as people who avoided the vitamin.

Despite the fact that vitamin C couldn't keep colds away entirely, the tests could not be called a total failure. When the researchers added up the total days that the subjects in the study were sick, and they examined the number and severity of their cold symptoms, they found that those who took vitamin C were not sick as severely or as long as those who did not take vitamins.

Some skeptics insisted on proclaiming vitamin C a failure against colds, and others pointed out that its proven effectiveness in frequently curtailing cold symptoms meant that it did more against the cold than almost all the so-called cold remedies available over the counter. In addition, the possible side effects of vitamin C are a lot milder than many of the ineffective cold remedies that people take.

Will vitamin C work for you? The researchers found it does not seem to help everyone in their battle against colds, but in some people the vitamin enables them to recover more quickly from this uncomfortable malady.

Q: Can nursing mothers follow a vegetarian diet and still produce breast milk that contains all the necessary vitamins?

A: To make sure they are getting sufficient vitamins and that these vitamins are in their breast milk, all nursing mothers should take a multivitamin. Vegetarians who nurse must be especially careful to take a supplement that contains the RDA for vitamin B_{12}, a nutrient that is not found in vegetarian foods (it is found in milk and eggs). Lack of this vitamin can lead to pernicious anemia, a condition producing irreversible damage to the nervous system. You should also consult your pediatrician for a liquid multivitamin you can give your baby.

There has been at least one documented case where a vegetarian nursing mother who did not take a supplement produced breast milk lacking B_{12}. This occurred even though tests of her blood levels for the vitamin indicated that she had adequate amounts in her body, but the vitamin was not getting into her milk and her baby became seriously ill until injections of B_{12} were administered.

Some people in other parts of the world may be able to make vitamin B_{12} for themselves. Tests of the intestinal bacteria of vegetarians living in India have indicated that the microorganisms they harbor can produce this nutrient. Vegetarians living in western Europe and the United States do not seem to possess bacteria with this ability. For some unexplained reason, after Indian vegetarians move to a Western country, their bacteria apparently lose this nutrient-producing ability. Consequently, many of these migrants have suffered vitamin B_{12} deficiency.

If you have reason to worry about your B_{12} status, ask your doctor to test your blood levels. If they are below normal or in what is called the low-normal range, you will probably need to take supplements.

Q: When you eat junk food, does it destroy vitamins in your body?

A: While junk food—refined food high in sugar and fat—does not directly destroy the vitamins in your body, there is evidence that it can help use them up. Foods high in refined sugar, for instance, often lack the vitamins and minerals that are used as coenzymes in the metabolic processes that absorb, transport, store, and burn the sugars and other carbohydrates that you consume in your diet. After you eat a sugary food, your body has to muster the necessary substances for these duties from other sources. Since the sugary food does not contribute any of the nutrients necessary for these processes, it can be said to aid in their depletion.

Q: Should you take vitamins that also contain iron? I've been told that supplements with iron will give you more energy.

A: Recent studies seem to indicate that taking supplementary iron is not a good idea for most healthy people. The only individuals who almost always should take iron in their supplements are pregnant women.

Although iron is necessary to prevent anemia, a condition characterized by weakness, pale skin, and shortness of breath, too much iron may be just as bad or worse for you than not enough. If you are not anemic, but merely feel weak and lacking energy much of the time, iron supplements will probably not restore your personal energy. In either case, if you suspect you suffer from anemia or if you have a serious problem with gathering the strength to lead a satisfyingly full life, you should consult a physician.

In Third World countries where malnutrition is a serious and widespread problem, iron deficiency is rampant, but in the United States and other developed countries, researchers have begun to turn up evidence that a surplus of iron in our diets may be contributing to heart disease and cancer. One study of heart disease victims revealed elevated iron levels in their blood. Research in Sweden showed that ten years after the amount of iron in fortified flour was doubled, liver cancer among women more than tripled.

If you are concerned about your iron intake, instead of taking iron supplements, slightly increase your consumption of lean meats and fish. The iron in meats is absorbed very efficiently and unknown food factors in meat will also increase your iron absorption from vegetables. To improve your absorption of iron from strictly vegetarian meals, take vitamin C with each meal or consume foods such as orange juice that are high in vitamin C. This vitamin enhances iron absorption from vegetarian sources.

You can also increase iron absorption by avoiding coffee or tea with vegetarian meals. The tannins in these drinks will inhibit iron absorption. Do not eat a diet extremely high in fiber, since fiber may tie up iron in the digestive system and cause it to be eliminated. (This effect has not been completely proven to everyone's satisfaction.)

Q: I believe that vitamins make me feel better and keep me from suffering the terrible winter colds I used to get, but they're expensive. Is it worth it to spend $20 a month on vitamins for myself?

A: You may be spending a little too much, but if you add up the health benefits of vitamins, you'll find that they are a health bargain compared to the costs of medicine you might be taking if you were to get sick. Considering the preventive attributes of antioxidant vitamins C and E and beta-carotene, which can help prevent cancer and heart disease; the way vitamin C shortens and alleviates the symptoms of colds; the possible way folate can protect against birth defects; and the benefits to your immune system from getting adequate vitamins; these helpful nutrients are well worth the price. Just compare their cost to one trip to the doctor's office.

With all that in mind, there may be ways you can hold down the cost of your vitamins. Try taking a store brand of multivitamin instead of a more expensive, heavily advertised private brand. Make sure the store brand is from an outfit with a nationally recognized reputation. Instead of taking multivitamins with high levels of vitamin C and E, which can be very pricy, purchase these nutrients separately. They do not cost that much.

Do not buy specialized formulations advertised as effective against stress or specially concocted for athletes. These may be more expensive, but they generally do not contain different ingredients than normal multivitamins, or, if they do, they will contain nutrients you do not really need. To hold down costs, avoid the expensive multivitamins that require you to take more than one pill or tablet daily. The vitamins you take several times a day may help you absorb your vitamins more completely, but you pay for the privilege.

According to the Center for Science in the Public Interest, if you spend more than $10 a month on all of your vitamins, you are paying too much. On the other hand, if you have found a combination of supplements that keep you feeling in excellent health, they are probably worth whatever you pay for them.

Q: I've been told that riboflavin is used to treat boric acid poisoning. Should I keep it in my medicine chest so I can use it in emergencies?

A: While riboflavin (vitamin B_2) is sometimes used to offset the effects of ingesting boric acid, you should never attempt to treat this condition by yourself. In case of accidental poisonings, you should always call your local poison control center, a hospital emergency room, or your doctor. Immediate professional help is crucial. Identify the poison to the person you reach on the phone and follow their instructions.

14

Guide to Other Types of Nutrient Supplements

Fiber

The 1970s were an expansive decade for nutrition scientists and supplement marketers. As one group of researchers near the Arctic Circle was discovering the benefits of fish oil in the Eskimo diet, another group farther south, in Africa, was investigating the benefits of fiber. Both discoveries would lead to important insights into how nutrition affects human health. They would also provide the scientific rationale for the creation of lucrative new supplements, fish oil capsules and fiber pills, both of which would bring in added revenues for nutrient marketers.

The fiber researchers certainly didn't start their work with supplements in mind. They were trying to understand why the diseases that beset Africans were so different from those suffered by West Europeans and Americans. In 1974, Dr. Denis Burkitt thought he had the answer, and that year he published a study concluding that it was the fiber in their diet that kept rural Africans from suffering the digestive diseases common among people living in urban areas.

It wasn't long after this study appeared that the

original fiber supplements, bran flakes, began to be heavily promoted as the cure-all for a long list of digestive diseases and conditions including constipation and diverticulitis. Capsules filled with "fiber" were soon to follow.

The Complexities of Fiber

While fiber should be a large part of the healthy diet that accompanies your vitamin supplementation, fiber supplements are too expensive and inefficient to be a central part of an optimal health plan. Fiber supplements just can't do justice to the complex part of our diet classified as fiber. Because of fiber's complexity and variety, the mere addition of bran flakes or a fiber pill to the usual fiber-poor American diet will not produce significant health benefits. It is a drastic oversimplification to think that a single type of fiber such as that found in a few daily fiber capsules will be able to supply you with a sufficient amount or variety of fiber.

The very word *fiber* is misleading, implying that all fiber is similar and can be grouped together under one heading. As the research on fiber since 1974 has shown, fiber consists of many different substances, few of which are well-understood by nutrition scientists. Just as vitamins are divided into two main groups (fat-soluble and water-soluble vitamins) the many varieties of fiber also fall under two main headings, water-solube and water-insoluble fiber.

Fiber Is Only in Vegetables

All fibers are found only in vegetarian foods. Neither soluble nor insoluble fibers can be processed by the enzymes in your digestive tract. This indigestibility was the reason why, until the 1970s, nutritionists didn't attach much importance to fiber. How important could fiber be to health, they thought, if this substance emerged relatively intact after traveling the length of your digestive system? When refined foods such as white bread and white rice originally had their fiber removed, no one thought it mattered. These were considered improved foods because digestion of their protein and other nutrients wouldn't be hindered by the presence of indigestible fiber.

Now, of course, we know that just because fiber passes through us without being absorbed, it still has important implications for our health and nutrition. For one thing, although fiber is not digested, it engages in many reactions as it passes through us. Soluble fiber forms a gelatinous mass as it wends its way through the gut and by so doing helps produce a softer stool. Soluble fiber also reacts with chemicals in food, binding them and making them pass out of the body rather than being absorbed. The soluble fibers that perform this function include substances called pectins and gums, which are contained in significant quantity in oats, citrus fruits, and apples. Keep in mind, however, that these and all vegetarian foods are a complex combination of many different fiber varieties.

Insoluble fibers expand like sponges in the digestive tract, soaking up large amounts of water, softening stools but also increasing the size of stools and speeding their elimination. In contrast to the soluble fibers, which are mostly formed from the inner structures of the cells in fruits and vegetables, insoluble fibers derive from the cell walls of vegetarian foods. These fibers include substances called lignin, cellulose, and hemicellulose and are found largely in cereal brans, whole grains, legumes (beans, peanuts, lentils), seeds, and fruits.

Disappearing Fiber

Because of the popularity of refined foods, the amount of fiber in our diets has steadily dropped during the past hundred years. Scientists have found that our fiber intake is less than half of that consumed by many people of the Third World. The most obvious medical problem associated with our meager fiber intake is constipation. Insoluble fibers, in particular, mitigate constipation by softening stools and enlarging them, processes that make them speed through the digestive tract. In addition, the bacteria population of your intestines feed on these fibers and produce a mixture of chemicals that also speeds their elimination.

In the absence of insoluble fiber, little water is retained in stools and they shrink and harden, making them difficult to pass. Straining to eliminate these stools can cause or exacerbate hemorrhoids and high blood pressure.

Lack of fiber also worsens a condition called diverticulitis, a condition characterized by the formation of small pouches in the walls of the intestestines. It is estimated that in the United States about one in three people over the age of fifty suffer diverticulitis to some degree. When these pouches become inflamed and painful because of trapped waste material, diverticulitis grows painful. Fiber can be instrumental in treating this condition, although it can't completely cure it.

Another intestinal problem, irritable bowel syndrome (IBS), can be helped by fiber. This condition occurs when the lower intestine contracts, causing diarrhea, pain, and gas. Some experts blame IBS at least partly on the consumption of a refined diet and recommend increases in fibrous foods to combat the syndrome.

Fiber and Heart Disease

Soluble fiber has received a great deal of publicity for its possible effectiveness in preventing heart disease. Research indicates that the soluble fiber in oat bran, legumes, and vegetables can lower LDL cholesterol (the kind that oxidizes and forms harmful plaque in arteries) without dropping your blood level of HDLs (the cholesterol that keeps plaque from forming). The insoluble fibers in foods such as wheat bran do not have this effect.

The mechanism for soluble fiber's cholesterol benefit is not known. Some scientists theorize that bile acids, the chemicals used to form cholesterol, may react with soluble fiber and be eliminated from the body with them instead of being absorbed in the blood, or the fiber may interact with certain enzymes responsible for cholesterol regulation. In any case, eating plenty of oats, lentils, and beans can improve your cholesterol profile.

Fiber Fights Colon Cancer

Comparisons of the U.S. population, which eats little fiber and lots of meat, with countries that eat a great deal of fiber and fewer animal products seem to show that as dietary fiber increases, colon cancer decreases. Although some experts say these studies don't prove a direct relationship between fiber and colon cancer (the people in fiber-eating countries may be doing something else that prevents colon cancer) researchers have shown that the insoluble fiber in wheat bran can help shrink intestinal polyps, precancerous growths that almost always increase in size and often prove fatal.

Here, too, no one has been able to figure out how fiber does its magic. In working against colon cancer, the second most common cancer in the United States, fiber may be effective because it moves stools out faster, giving carcinogenic chemicals less time to react with the intestinal walls before they are eliminated, or it may bind with these cancer-causing villains, turning them into substances no longer carcinogenic.

Fiber Helps Diabetics

If scientists still scratch their heads over how fiber can benefit cholesterol levels, they are downright stumped over its ability to moderate blood levels of sugar, a major concern of diabetics. Research at the University of Kentucky has demonstrated that diets high in fiber and other carbohydrates can help diabetics cut back on the insulin they are required to take. At the same time, fiber also improves glucose tolerance. Whether these benefits are caused by fiber's action in restricting glucose absorption or in slowing the movement of food from the stomach to the intestines after a meal or some other interaction, is not clear, but it is now recommended that diabetics eat fibrous foods.

Pills Versus Food

To get the full benefits of fiber, you must eat a wide variety of vegetarian foods. Too little is known about the different kinds of fibers to recommend one particular food or supplement. Although some fiber supplements promise they can help you lose weight by filling you up on few calories (fiber, since it is not digested, contains zero calories), eating fibrous foods can fill you up more than a pill can, and you'll take in other nutritive factors besides fiber.

Another problem with fiber pills is that they don't contain all that much fiber. For instance, a pill that contains a gram of fiber has less than half the fiber of an apple. That's hardly a bargain. The apple will also contain vitamins and minerals, as well as many more types of fiber than are in the pill, and it will be more satisfying to consume.

Fiber's Interaction With Vitamins

Some people are concerned that eating a high-fiber diet will hinder their vitamin absorption. Since fiber in the digestive tract can tie up some nutrients and make them pass out of the body, it's been suggested that fiber eliminates vitamins and makes less of them available for the body's use.

Despite these fears, unless you are on the brink of serious malnourishment, you probably have nothing to fear from fiber. The studies indicating that fiber interferes with nutrient absorption were originally performed on chickens. That research showed that chickens fed a diet of soybeans did not grow normally. The cause was phytate, a chemical in soy and some other high-fiber foods that interferes with zinc absorption. There also have been other studies showing that very high fiber intakes could theoretically interfere with calcium and iron absorption in the body.

Outside of the lab and the chicken farm, however, no one has shown that boosting your fiber intake will hurt your vitamin or mineral profile significantly. Phytate is not in all fibrous foods. It's missing in most vegetables. When foods with phytate are baked (as whole wheat is baked when made into bread), the phytate is largely broken down.

Consequently, fiber should be an integral part of your optimal health plan: Eat plenty of green vegetables. For main courses have legumes, which contain ample amounts of protein as well as fiber. For dessert, have a piece of fruit. For breakfast, eat high-fiber cereals such as oatmeal and whole wheat squares. You'll be doing your health a favor.

Fish Oil

Omega 3 fatty acids are a type of fat that has been the subject of recent study by nutrition scientists, and they are found primarily in fish. It is believed that this family of fats, which technically are designated as long-chain polyunsaturated fatty acids, can cut your risk of heart disease.

The idea that fish fat or some other nutritive substance in fish could protect against cardiovascular disease has been around since the 1940s. At that time a British doctor, Hugh Sinclair, observed that Eskimos who ate tremendous amounts of fish, seals, whale meat, and other animal fats from seagoing creatures had a remarkably low incidence of cardiovascular disease despite the fact that they ate no fruits and vegetables at all. At the time he made these observations, Sinclair was ignored or written of as an obsessed eccentric. Most western nutrition scientists in those years were focused on how vegetarian diets could lower the risk of heart disease.

It wasn't until the 1970s that other researchers began to take seriously the idea that something the Eskimos were eating were keeping their arteries clear and their hearts healthy. At that time, Danish scientists performed detailed analyses of the blood of men in Denmark and compared it to Eskimo blood. All the subjects of the study ate high-fat diets. The Eskimos had significantly lower triglyceride and LDL levels (both of which are markers indicating risk of heart disease) than the Danes. At the same time, the Eskimos had higher levels of

HDL, the type of cholesterol that protects against heart disease.

Fish Fat Influences Prostaglandins

The researchers eventually traced at least part of the Eskimos' high-fat diet's effect on cardiovascular health to its influence on prostaglandins, chemical messengers that determine many different body functions including how quickly blood clots. In particular, the omega 3 fatty acids in the diet were found to increase the production of prostacyclin, a prostaglandin that prolongs clotting time. It apparently does this by changing the chemical constituents of platelets, cells in the blood that collect and form a blood clot wherever a blood vessel is injured.

Because they eat so many omega 3 fatty acids and their platelets are slow to form clots, Eskimos, when cut, bleed for a relatively long time. For instance, while a cut that you might suffer would stop bleeding in less than five minutes, a comparable injury to an Eskimo would probably bleed for longer than eight minutes.

While blood clots are useful for keeping us from bleeding to death every time we injure ourselves, they can be dangerous when clumps of platelets gather inside blood vessels and block blood flow, causing serious medical problems. By reducing the tendency of platelets to stick together, fish oils reduce the risk of a blood clot forming in a dangerous, life-threatening location such as a coronary artery, where it could bring on a heart attack, or in a blood vessel supplying the brain, where it can cause a stroke.

Fish Oil Supplements

In contrast to the indifference that greeted Dr. Sinclair's original discovery of the Eskimos' resistance to heart disease in the 1940s, the further scientific work on this phenomenon and the investigation into the benefits of fish oil in the 1970s and 1980s was celebrated with the massive marketing of fish oil supplements. Today, millions of dollars worth of omega 3 capsules have been sold and continue to sell. Most of these capsules contain a particular fatty acid known as eicosapentanoic acid (EPA).

Are fish oil capsules really a healthy best buy? There's no easy answer to this question. The experts are still arguing over their alleged benefits. According to the opposing points of view, these supplements are either the perfect addition to your vitamin supplementation program or a waste of money that can introduce dangerous chemicals into your diet.

As more research on these substances becomes available, it is beginning to look like the naysayers are right. Although there's evidence to believe that omega 3 fatty acids may someday be used to prevent heart disease, fight arthritis, and boost immunity, the usefulness of taking fish oil capsules in their present form is still too uncertain to be recommended.

The Problems With Fish Oil

Even the marketers of fish oil capsules recognize that these supplements, by themselves, are no panacea for health problems. It is generally agreed that if you take these capsules but do not change other lifestyle habits, you will not become as impervious to heart disease as an Eskimo. For instance, fish oil capsules won't offset the negative health effects of eating a diet high in red meat and not getting any exercise. Traditional Eskimos don't mix double cheeseburgers with their whale meat.

It is also evident that you have to take a great many fish oil capsules to get the same amount of omega 3 fatty acids that an Eskimo might consume—anywhere from twelve to thirty capsules a day. That kind of massive intake of fish oil capsules could have long-term consequences that no one knows about. Taking dozens of capsules is not the same as eating a diet of Arctic fish and whales. Few studies have been performed measuring what happens to you when you take very many of these capsules for a long time, so those kinds of doses could be risky.

There are other potential hazards to these supplements. When you down a fish oil capsule, you don't only swallow omega 3 fatty acids, you also may be getting a very high dose of vitamins A and D, nutrients that can be toxic in large amounts. Added to that danger, consuming fish oil can cause your body to become deficient in vitamin E. To offset this possibility, many capsule makers have begun adding vitamin E to their capsules.

There may also be other chemicals in the capsules besides those already mentioned. Together with those fat-soluble vitamins, you may be swallowing pesticides and other substances that the fish accumulated in swims through polluted water. This is especially likely to occur if the fish oil has been extracted from fish livers, the organ that filters out contaminants from the fish's environment.

Let Them Eat Fish

Most of the large studies that have established the benefit of fish oil have measured fish consumption, not the swallowing of fish oil capsules. Fourteen years of research in Stockholm that looked at about 11,000 identical twins found that the twins who ate the most fish had a much lower risk of dying from heart attacks than those who hardly ever ate fish.

A Dutch study that looked at the eating habits of more than 800 men reported similar results. In this research, which covered a period of twenty years, men who ate more than 30 grams of fish a day had half the chance of dying from heart disease than those who eschewed seafood.

While fish oil advocates point to studies like this to support their claims for fish oil capsules, it's important to note that this research measured fish consumption, not capsule consumption. In particular, the Dutch study recommended consuming an average of 30 grams of fish a day, an amount that comes out to just about an ounce. In comparison, Eskimos daily eat about a pound of fish and other meat from seagoing animals. The Dutch researchers recommended merely eating two fish dishes a week to get the healthy heart benefits from fish.

Admittedly, by eating fish instead of taking fish oil capsules, you'll get a lot less omega 3 fatty acids than do Eskimos, but as you can see, the studies show that you don't have to eat a lot of fish to benefit your heart. Two cans of tuna a week seem to be enough.

The final argument against taking fish oil supplements is the paucity of information about what else there might be in fish that benefits health. It could be that there are other unknown factors besides the oils that are the causes of the benefits shown in these studies. If there are health factors in fish, fish oil capsules probably do not contain them.

15

Don't Let Your Diet Defeat Your Vitamin Program

Eating the Right Diet

It is a mistake to think that vitamin supplements or any other kind of nutrients that come in pills can fully compensate for a diet and lifestyle that incorporate poor health habits. Nutrient supplements may be able to fill in some of the sketchy corners of your diet, where you may occasionally not be eating enough of the right foods for all the nutrients you need, and a good helping of the antioxidants can lower your risk of disease, but your diet has to be the foundation of your optimal health plan.

An optimal diet is not hard to describe. It should emphasize a wide variety of vegetarian foods and go easy on the sugar, fat, and salt. Eating this type of diet seems to be an elusive goal for many of us. We delight in fried foods, thick steaks, and sweet desserts. Of course, there's nothing wrong with indulging our taste buds within moderation. Consistent overindulgence is what seems to lead our diets astray.

Sugar, the Ultimate Empty Calorie

The phrase *empty calorie* is one of those clichés that slips off the tongues of many but is fully understood by few. Consequently, many so-called nutrition experts advocate cutting the empty calories of sugar out of your diet and eating more complex carbohydrates as though a complex carbohydrate were inherently healthier than the simpler carbohydrates.

Actually, complex carbohydrates should make up the major part of a healthy diet because of the vitamins, minerals, fiber, and other food factors that usually accompany them in food. Even though many people think that complex carbohydrates in and of themselves are desirable nutrients, these carbohydrates are merely long chains of simple sugars. When you eat complex carbohydrates, these chains, known as polysaccharides, are quickly broken down into sugar in the digestive tract. The true benefits of complex carbohydrates are the company they keep, other nutrients you consume with them when you eat foods such as legumes (beans, lentils), grains, vegetables, and cereals. Alone, complex carbohydrates are probably no better for you than the simple carbohydrates that make up the links in their chains.

Of course, it is this isolation from other nutrients that gives sugar the title *empty calorie*. As a matter of fact, the only thing refined sugar provides is calories, but in our daily lives we rarely eat the totally empty calories of straight sugar. Unfortunately, we usually consume the sweet stuff with significant amounts of fat.

This combination of sugar and fat represented by such popular foods as ice cream, candy bars, cakes, and cookies can be dangerous to your health for several reasons, the chief one being its tendency to make you fatter. Obesity is one of America's major health problems and has been linked to causing or worsening a long list of illnesses from diabetes to cancer to heart disease. If you are looking for optimal health from vitamins, keeping your weight down by avoiding overindulgences in sugary and fatty foods should be a basic component of your health program.

Sweet Tooth or Fat Tooth?

Be warned: It may not be very easy to hold back on the fat when you eat the typical American diet. Although a myth about sugar claims that many of us are addicted to sugar's sweet taste, and it is a craving for sugar that often causes overeating, the truth is that it is usually sugar's combination with fat in many foods that causes many people to lose control of their appetites and eat too much. Although many people believe that they have a sweet tooth—a propensity to pig out on sugary foods— most often it is the high level of fat in our diets that causes folks to overindulge.

As Adam Drewnowski, Ph.D., head of the human nutrition department of the University of Michigan, puts it, "What many people call a sweet tooth should really be called a fat tooth." While you may think that it is the sweet taste of candy bars, cookies, cakes, pies, and donuts that tempts you into stuffing yourself, it is the fat, or the combination of sugar and fat, that is so alluring to the taste buds and makes you overindulge.

Sugar adds fattening calories to your diet in terms of calories per weight of food, but fat almost always adds more. A close examination of many sweet foods shows that those sweets often contain more fat calories than sugar calories. As a general rule, for every gram of sugar you consume, your body will liberate about 4 calories. The same amount of fat, however, contains 9 calories, more than twice as many as sugar.

The fattening power of fat, as opposed to sugar, doesn't stop at the mere calorie content. It has also been shown that fat calories are more fattening than sugar. In other words, the calories in sugar are not as easily converted into fat cells by the human body as are the calories in fat.

There's more bad news: According to studies done on animals in Japan, diets that combine fats and sugar at each meal are probably even more fattening than diets with the same amounts of calories in which the fatty and sugary foods are eaten at separate times. (The physiological explanation for this phenomenon has not yet been discovered.) If you eat a food like pizza oozing great gobs of fatty cheese and drink a soda at the same meal, the combined effect of the cheese and sugar in the soda may make you gain more weight than if you waited to drink the soda later. The same fattening synergistic effect is caused by consumption of a burger with fries and a sugary soft drink.

That said, how does one go about determining how much sugar is in your diet and what you should do about it? A good place to start is with limiting soft drinks. According to the Food and Drug Administration, the average male between twelve and twenty-nine years of age downs two cans of sugar-sweetened soda pop a day, while women of that age drink one and a half cans daily. Because there are 10 teaspoons of sugar dissolved in each can of soda, American men and boys are taking in an average of 20 teaspoons of sugar a day from their soda drinking alone. Women are consuming 15 teaspoons.

Strategies for controlling your calories include switching from high-fat ice cream to low-fat or nonfat ice milk or frozen yogurt. Then, instead of regular pizza with your soda, try pizza with reduced cheese or, if you want to lessen the effect of having sugar and fat together, have a glass of water with your pizza instead of a cup of soda with its large dose of sugar.

High in Fructose Means Trouble

If you are looking for an optimal diet to go along with your vitamin supplements, it is probably a good idea to stay away from soft drinks altogether. A troubling aspect to the sugar in soda pop is the fact that it is often present in the form of high-fructose corn syrup, a substance derived from corn but with significantly different characteristics than conventional corn syrup. As its name implies, high-fructose corn syrup contains much more fructose than other sweeteners. Although fructose is sometimes referred to as fruit sugar, this is really a misnomer. Fructose is merely one of the several types of sugar found in fruits.

Because this corn by-product is so economical compared to other sweeteners, food companies have been increasing their use of high-fructose corn syrup in packaged foods. Studies done by the U.S. Department of Agriculture indicate that this food additive can raise your serum cholesterol (the cholesterol in your blood) when it is consumed with a diet high in saturated fat and cholesterol. Many Americans eat just such a diet. Consequently, their consumption of this variety of corn syrup in sodas, sauces, breakfast cereals, breads, and other foods may be increasing their risk of heart disease. The research into this subject has not revealed just how fructose adversely effects blood cholesterol, but the studies have shown that consuming this type of syrup raises cholesterol more than a comparable amount of cornstarch does.

Despite the possible risk from eating high-fructose corn syrup, which is actually a combination of the sugars glucose and fructose, you probably consume a lot more of this sweetener than you used to. Statistics demonstrate that the average American ate about 5 pounds of high-fructose corn syrup a year back in the mid-1970s. By the latter part of the 1980s, we were each consuming 45 pounds. Today, we are probably taking in even more. Researchers who have looked into this additive caution that no one has any idea what the long-term health effects of eating this tremendous amount of fructose will be.

Besides the unknown long-term effects of fructose consumption, you should watch out for fructose's short-term consequences. In the human digestive tract, fructose takes a fairly long time to be digested compared to other sugars and starches (starches are chains of simple sugars). Some people seem to have trouble digesting fructose and they can develop indigestion, stomachaches, and diarrhea when they eat a great deal of this sugar.

If you think you have this problem, check food labels and limit your consumption of foods that list high-fructose corn syrup or fructose among their prime ingredients. Be especially careful to limit how much soda you drink, since soft drinks are a prime source of this nutrient.

The Blood Sugar Myth

A misconception about sugar is that eating it will make you feel great for a few moments and then quickly let you crash after it is absorbed into your body. Proponents of this myth argue that downing sugar rapidly boosts blood sugar levels, making you feel alert, but then boomerangs when blood sugar levels drop along with your spirits.

The truth is that the phenomenon of the blood sugar rush is a complicated, murky physiological event that is not easily explained and that is probably not due to the consumption of pure sugar. Some foods do boost blood sugar faster than others, but it is not intuitively obvious which foods do this, and researchers have not been able to discern clear mechanisms that would explain why some foods send blood sugar up rapidly while others have a slower, more sluggish effect.

For instance, a study at the University of Toronto demonstrated that foods rich in carbohydrates such as potatoes (no butter) and plain bread (hold the cream cheese), will usually raise your blood sugar much more quickly than will a candy bar. Why does this happen? No one has a ready answer, although some suspect that the fat in the candy bar may retard the body's absorption of sugar and thereby slow the rise in blood sugar levels.

There are other complicating factors. The other foods you eat at a single meal or snack also affect how fast your body absorbs the sugar you consume. On top of that, how the food is prepared—fried, microwaved, sautéed, diced, etc.—influences how it is taken into the body. To say that eating a simple sugar like sucrose (table sugar) will bounce your blood sugar up and then drag it down is an oversimplification. Foods rich in starch and not necessarily sugar can have that same effect.

All Sugars Are Equal

Speaking of various types of sugars, what about the idea that some sugar is better for you than others? Aren't foods like honey, molasses, and brown sugar more natural and better for you than other forms of sugar such as highly refined white sugar? Aside from the fact no one agrees on the precise definition of *natural,* there is no scientific evidence to support the idea that any form of sugar is better for the human body than any other. Molasses and honey contain some minerals,

but probably not enough to affect your health one way
or another.

Don't believe that brown sugar is a less refined food
than white sugar, either. In many cases, the brown sugar
you consume is merely white sugar with a coloring such
as caramel added to give it a dark color.

Sugar Hides the Fat

Another way sugar can mislead you is when it is added
to recipes and foods to make it seem as though the level of
fat in food is lower than it really is. During the past few
years, much has been made of the fact that heart-healthy
diets should derive about 55 to 60 percent of their calories
from carbohydrates, which includes sugar, and only about
30 percent or less of their calories from fat. As a result,
some foods and recipes contain extra amounts of sugar
(simple carbohydrate) to lower the apparent percentage
of calories coming from fat, but these foods still contain
the same amount of fat. The addition of sugar only makes
it seem relatively less.

Artificial Sweetener

If the simple sugar in soda pop provides undesirable
calories, does drinking diet soda flavored with aspartame
convey any health benefits? Don't count on it. Despite the
fact that foods containing aspartame have been marketed
as part of a "healthy lifestyle," no health benefits have
been scientifically linked to this sweetener.

Although aspartame, most frequently marketed under
the brand name NutraSweet, has enjoyed explosive sales
growth and popularity during the past few years, drinking
soft drinks flavored with aspartame or eating foods that

use aspartame instead of sugar is no guarantee that you will shed or keep off unwanted pounds. Only if you cut your dietary calories and/or increase your physical activity, will you lose and keep off weight. That is true, whether or not you consume so-called diet foods such as diet soft drinks.

Sugar in Moderation

Since some sugar in the diet is unavoidable, the best advice is to consume this family of chemicals in moderation. As long as you eat a prudent low-fat diet with healthy doses of fiber-filled vegetarian foods, take your vitamins, and get enough exercise, indulging in the sweet stuff now and then probably won't hurt, but don't think that vitamins, exercise, or any other kind of health regimen will make up for a poor diet that includes excess sugar. For optimal health, cut back on your sugar and take your vitamin supplements.

Watch the Fat

If you never ate another ounce of sugar in your life, you could survive quite nicely getting all your carbo-hydrates from starches. You cannot say the same kind of thing about fat. Even though many nutrition-minded people consider fat to be as much of a dietary villain as sugar, you would not live very long on a totally fat-free diet. Your body needs fat to make hormones, chemical messengers that travel through the blood. Even though the average American eats enough fat to implicate this nutrient in causing our high rates of obesity, cancer, and heart disease, it is a mistake to try to eliminate fat from your diet completely.

Dietary fat enables your body to properly absorb the fat-soluble vitamins A, E, and D. For instance, research has shown that taking a vitamin E supplement along with a meal that contains a modicum of fat allows your body to take in a lot more vitamin E from the vitamin capsule than when you take this vitamin on an empty stomach or after a meal or snack that is very low or completely lacking in fat. This is an excellent example of how vitamin supplements and your diet have a synergistic effect on your nutrition and health. You should never mindlessly pop vitamin supplements without paying attention to your diet.

Of course, the fact that fat helps you absorb extra vitamins from your food and vitamin pills is not a license to eat whatever fat you want. It's especially not a good reason to indulge in the kinds of fats that are most heavily advertised and marketed on television and in popular magazines, the fats in candy and margarine. The fats in those foods can be detrimental to your heart.

Fattening Fat

Ounce for ounce, fat of any kind is the most fattening nutrient that you can eat. By weight it has more than twice the number of calories of protein or carbohydrate. Studies show that people who eat the most fat generally weigh the most. When you eat sugar and fat together, as noted before, the combination is especially fattening.

Besides its calories, fat has some special physiological tricks of its own that make it dangerous to your waistline. A study at the Stanford University School of Medicine demonstrated that the amount of fat in men's diets correlated with how overweight they were. The mere number of calories they reported eating had no apparent statistical effect on the amount of body fat they carried around tucked behind their belts. Only the fat seemed to matter.

Consequently, the researchers at Stanford believe that fat's ability to make us fatter at least partly accounts for the fact that although we eat more than 3 percent fewer calories than did Americans in 1900, the percentage of overweight citizens has zoomed up dramatically in the last few decades. Our meals today contain a third more fat than they did back in the horse and carriage days.

The fact that we eat less food, however, also means that we take in fewer vitamins in our diet than we used to. Also, our food is so much more thoroughly processed and refined than the food we ate in 1900, which further depletes our diets of both vitamins and fiber. Put these facts together—more fat, fewer nutrients—and you can see why the foods we eat are probably contributing to the rise in the rates of heart disease and cancer.

Fatty Food Makes Fat Stomachs

Every calorie of dietary fat you eat is more likely to end up as body fat than the calories of carbohydrate you consume. When fat is absorbed from your digestive tract and then transported to your fat cells to be stashed as cellulite or in your potbelly, less than 5 percent of the fat calories are used up and burned in the fat storing process. In contrast, when carbohydrates are utilized for the same purpose, up to 25 percent of the carbohydrate calories are consumed in the process.

That means that you can chow down on a lot more high-carbohydrate food than fatty food without risking obesity. For instance, when you eat 100 calories of fat-rich food (about 10 grams, the amount in a tablespoon of butter or a cookie) you end up with about 95 of those calories actually becoming body fat, but 100 calories of carbohydrates (25 grams of food, the amount in a medium-size baked potato) only results in 75 calories becoming body fat.

Eating fat also does not raise your metabolic rate very much. Your metabolic rate is the rate at which your body uses up calories, and it increases after each meal. That's one reason why diet specialists advise eating many small meals during the day to keep your weight down. Every snack stokes your calorie furnace. If you fast or spend a long time between meals, the metabolic rate at which you burn calories drops, and when you eat a meal high in fat, your metabolic rate does not climb as high as it does after you eat carbohydrate foods.

Keep Your Weight Down

If you are looking to vitamins to aid your health, your optimal supplement program will include dietary measures that keep your weight down. Letting yourself gain weight while taking extra vitamins is counterproductive. The extra fat on your body creates an internal environment conducive to conditions like diabetes, cancer, and heart disease. It's only by maintaining a desirable weight while taking supplements and eating a low-fat diet that you can stay as healthy as possible.

The reason that fat is so alluring to the palate is due to its taste-enhancing abilities and the feeling of fullness it produces at the end of a meal or snack. The presence of fat actually produces a chemical reaction that helps the flavors of food react pleasurably with our taste buds. When spices are in food, fat helps release their flavors. Without fat, many foods taste dull and unrewarding. That's one reason why French fried potatoes are so much more popular than baked potatoes. The deep frying method of cooking French fries gives them a juicy feel and taste that plain baked potatoes, which lack the fat, can't match.

According to sensory experts who have studied how taste buds sense flavor, fat rounds off flavorings. Even though science has not satisfactorily explained how this occurs, in a metaphorical sense, fat makes food flavors taste bigger and rounder and more satisfying. Added to this, fat gives foods a more desirable mouth feel and texture. The feel of fat in your mouth soothes.

Fat also makes you feel comfortably full for a long time, because it sits in the digestive tract for a relatively extended period. While carbohydrates and proteins are efficiently digested and absorbed after a meal, fat can sit in the intestines for up to six hours. That means you won't be hungry too soon again after eating fatty foods.

Fat in Moderation

The advice sounds contradictory. On the one hand, Americans eat too much fat and must cut back, but on the other hand, fat is necessary for bodily functions and the absorption of fat-soluble vitamins, so you shouldn't cut it out entirely. What's the best course of action?

In the eyes of some experts, the main emphasis for most of us has to be on cutting back on fat. Today, Americans eat about 37 percent of their calories as fat. That's 7 percent too much fat, according the American Heart Association (AHA) and other organizations that believe we should be eating about 30 percent of our calories from fat. Other experts think even 30 percent is too high and that our dietary fat intake, for optimal health, should be down around 20 percent.

It's probably true that, for vitamins to do the most for your health, your diet should be around 20 percent or lower in fat. One reason the 30 percent figure is embraced by the AHA and others is that they just don't believe that you and I and our fellow Americans can eat 20 percent of our calories in fat. We're too hooked on French fries, steaks, fried chicken, burgers, and fast food to do it, they think. If they really thought we could hold back on the mayonnaise, which is virtually all fat, and the banana cream pies, they might advocate a 20 percent level of fat in the diet.

Of course, a big problem with proposing that we should eat 20 or even 30 percent of our calories as fat is that few people have any idea what this means. What does a diet that is 20 percent fat look like? How do you measure fat?

Rather than worry about the exact numbers governing the amount of fat in your diet, the best course of action is to eat a diet that emphasizes vegetables and vegetarian foods prepared with little or no fat. That means you should eat steamed or microwaved vegetables instead of frying or sautéeing them. If you boil them, use as little water as possible. The water will leach out a portion of the vitamins.

You can eat frozen vegetables as well as fresh. In some cases, frozen vegetables may even contain more vitamins than produce that has been sitting for days in the supermarket or your refrigerator. When you cook frozen vegetables, microwave them without adding water, even though frozen vegetable packages tell you to add water before microwaving. This will preserve more of the vitamins and will make the vegetables crunchier.

Vegetables almost always contain much less fat than meats and they usually contain vitamins such as beta-carotene and vitamin C that Americans don't get enough of. As a matter of fact, one nutritionist has claimed that if it weren't for the popularity of fast-food French fried potatoes, which contain a small amount of vitamin C, many Americans would have scurvy because they never eat any other food containing vitamin C.

Eat the Right Kinds of Fat

Vegetables have another dietary advantage. What little fat they contain is composed of unsaturated fats that are generally better for you than the saturated fats contained in meats and other animal products.

To talk about fats as saturated, unsaturated, polyunsaturated, or monounsaturated confuses many consumers. Even these general terms are an oversimplification of the fat situation. All fats are complex mixtures of substances known as fatty acids, the basic building blocks of fat. For example, the fat in butter is a combination of more than 500 different types of fatty acids.

Each fatty acid's classification as saturated, polyunsaturated, or monounsaturated depends on its chemical structure. The amount of saturation refers to the number of hydrogen atoms linked to the carbon atoms in the fatty acid. If all the available carbons are linked to hydrogens, the molecule is "saturated" with hydrogen; if two or more unsaturated bonds are available, the fatty acid is polyunsaturated; and if one bond has room for hydrogen, the acid is monounsaturated.

The easiest way to distinguish between saturated and unsaturated fats is by their solidity at room temperature. Fats that mostly contain saturated fatty acids, such as the fats on meat, are solids at room temperature. Mixtures of mostly unsaturated fatty acids, such as vegetable oils, are liquids.

A few years ago, the few vegetable fats that are highly saturated—palm oils and coconut oil—were virtually banned from our snack foods. At the time, several self-appointed public interest groups demanded that food companies take these fats out of cookies and cakes. Concerned about these oils' possible role in causing heart disease, these public interest groups used newspaper advertisements and letter writing campaigns to pressure food companies to find substitutes for these ingredients in desserts and convenience foods.

Palm and coconut oils, also known as tropical oils, had long been used in potato chips and cookies because of their taste, preservative quality, and the fact that they were solids at room temperature. Although these saturated oils are undesirable in a healthy diet, the amounts being consumed in convenience foods were relatively insignificant compared to the saturated fats we eat in our red meats and fried foods.

Nevertheless, bowing to the pressure and bad publicity (one notorious full-page newspaper ad referred to the "poisoning of America"), food companies stopped using tropical oils, much to the chagrin and indignation of farmers in Asia who had depended upon the U.S. market to sell the oils from their crops.

Our health was not helped by the tropical oil ban. The food companies have substituted different oils in cookies and cakes that may be more problematic than the oils they stopped using.

If you look at the typical label on a package of chocolate chip cookies, you will find that instead of tropical oils they now contain hydrogenated fat or oil. What this means is that in order to produce an acceptable cookie, the food manufacturer has used an unsaturated fat that has had hydrogen added.

By adding hydrogen, however, the food companies have also created fats that are probably just as unhealthy for you as saturated fats. Several studies have indicated that these hydrogenated fats, which are used in margarine to keep it solid at room temperature, are just as dangerous for your cardiovascular system as are saturated fats. Even though margarine companies have marketed their products for years as being healthier than butter, the accumulating scientific evidence shows that this almost certainly isn't so.

Sources of Saturated Fat in Your Diet

By far, the largest source of saturated fat in the American diet is still red meat. It has been estimated that about a third of our saturated fat is eaten in the form of foods such as burgers, steaks, ham, and London broil. Eating fish and chicken without the skin, which contains a large amount of fat, will reduce your intake of saturated fat. Better yet, eating mostly vegetarian foods will reduce your saturated fat intake even further. As a victim of heart disease, I have switched over completely to vegetarian foods in order to avoid saturated fats.

The next largest source of saturated fat consumed in the United States comes from whole milk and whole milk products such as cheese, ice cream, and yogurt. If you want to avoid the butterfat in milk, you should drink skim milk, which has almost no fat, and eat nonfat yogurt and cheeses. Of course, many people don't like the taste of milk products that have had the fat removed, but that is the only way to avoid milk's saturated fat. Drinking the so-called "1 percent" or "2 percent" milk will cut back your fat intake somewhat, but is not as effective as drinking nonfat milk.

Vegetable Oil and Cancer

The polyunsaturated fats in vegetable oils have several advantages over the saturated fat present in animal products. Polyunsaturated fatty acids (PUFAs) usually contain significant amounts of vitamin E, and they probably are less harmful to your cardiovascular system, but eating large amounts of PUFAs may be linked to the kinds of cancer that you take vitamin supplements to avoid.

Recent research indicates that consuming heavy doses of this oil in your food suppresses the immune system and keeps it from operating at optimum capacity. In scientific terms, PUFAs are said to have an immunosuppressive effect. In the laboratory, animals that are fed a diet overly rich in PUFAs have T cells (immune cells) that don't respond effectively to invasion by foreign substances or organisms. When researchers challenge the immune systems of these animals with skin grafts, their bodies have difficulty rejecting the foreign tissue.

Although scientists don't know how PUFAs depress the immune system's response to disease, it has been shown that this condition leads to an increased risk of breast cancer, prostate cancer, and colon cancer in animals.

Cut Back on Fat

You should limit your dietary fat of all kinds. Population studies comparing dietary fat eaten by humans support the research on fat that has been done on animals. For instance, while the rate of breast cancer is very low among Japanese women who live in Japan, when Japanese natives move to the United States and begin to consume an American-style high-fat diet, their breast cancer rate soon climbs to the usual American rate. Studies comparing breast cancer rates among various countries show that those populations consuming the highest amounts of fat generally have the highest breast cancer rates.

Population studies also demonstrate that colon cancer

rates vary with the amount of dietary fat that people eat. For example, Seventh Day Adventists, who eat a strictly vegetarian diet, have a lower rate of this disease than Americans who eat a diet high in animal fat.

As colon cancer develops, it is believed that a high-fat diet causes the bacteria in the lower intestine to produce higher levels of carcinogenic substances that speed the development of the disease. In addition, if a cancer victim eats a high-fat diet low in fiber, as is common in the U.S. diet, these carcinogenic substances remain longer in the lower intestine before being eliminated. The longer they stay in your body, the more harm they can do.

Monounsaturated Fat: The Healthiest Fat?

The one type of fat that gets the best press and the least approbation from dietitians and nutritionists are the monounsaturated fats, the kind of fat that predominates in olive oil, peanut oil, and canola oil.

The initial evidence that demonstrated the benefits of monounsaturated fats were studies of people who lived in the Mediterranean area, mostly Greeks and Italians, who ate diets high in fat but who enjoyed very low rates of heart disease. It was found that the olive oil they ate seemed to have a protective effect against cardiovascular problems.

The reason that diets whose fat mostly consists of monounsaturated fats seem to be better for your heart has to do with how the cholesterol in your blood is influenced by types and amounts of fat, as well as by the vitamins and other nutrients you ingest. In the section on vitamin C, we saw that diets high in vitamin C tend to lower your cholesterol. Generally speaking, the saturated fat in animal products raises the levels of harmful cholesterol in your blood, while the PUFAs are relatively neutral in relationship to cholesterol and the monounsaturates are beneficial.

When talking about cholesterol, it is important to distinguish between the cholesterol in your blood (also known as serum cholesterol) and the cholesterol in your food. Dietary cholesterol is only found in foods of animal origin. No vegetarian foods ever contain cholesterol, so when potato chips, cookies, cakes, or peanut butter trumpet the fact that they contain absolutely no cholesterol, they are merely reporting the fact that they are vegetarian foods.

However, a food can be cholesterol-free and still be harmful for your serum cholesterol. That's because the cholesterol you eat has only a limited influence on the cholesterol circulating in your blood. Your body produces its own cholesterol; it doesn't depend on the cholesterol it digests. Your blood cholesterol is more strongly affected by the saturated fat you consume than by the cholesterol in your food. For many of us, the more saturated fat we eat, the higher our cholesterol levels and the higher our risk of developing heart disease. This does not apply to everyone. Some people have a genetic resistance to developing heart disease no matter what diet they eat. At the present time, however, there is no reliable way to know if this applies to you.

Many experts now believe that while we should limit the fat in our diet, we can safely eat more monounsaturated fats than other types of fat. That's because monounsaturates help increase the amount of HDL, or good cholesterol, in our blood. HDLs help keep cholesterol from being deposited on artery walls. If, along with your vitamin supplement program, your diet contains relatively more monounsaturated fat than saturated or polyunsaturated fat, in other words, if it's heavy on the veggies and easy on the meat, the synergy between your healthy diet and extra vitamins should go a long way toward keeping your heart healthy and happy.

Protein Gets Great PR

While fat has long been vilified in the popular press as a nutritional villain, protein has enjoyed the reputation as a nutritional good guy. When most people think of protein, they think of muscle, since muscles are made of protein. From that association, it's a logical step to think that the more protein you eat, the more muscle you can grow, the better you'll look and feel. Therefore, massive amounts of dietary protein must be good for you. Right?

Not quite.

Although the word protein comes from a Greek term meaning *to win,* eating large quantities of protein or taking protein supplements doesn't create athletic champions or optimal health. As a matter of fact, if your diet persistently includes hefty portions of red meat, these protein-rich foods will probably slow you down instead of improving your athletic prowess.

True, protein is needed to build the muscles that we all admire on the millionaire athletes who grace televised sporting events, but a lot less is needed than most people assume should be consumed. Perfectly fine, bulging muscles can be built with the protein from vegetables. Meat and protein supplements are completely unnecessary.

Just as fats are made up of fatty acids, protein consists of chemicals called amino acids. When you eat protein, your body deconstructs the proteins into their constituent chains of amino acids and reconstructs them into your bodily infrastructure including your muscles, skin, kidneys, liver, and other organs and tissues. These amino acids also form the building blocks for hormones, enzymes, and blood cells. Just as there are only twenty-six letters in the English alphabet, but thousands of words can be made from these letters, so there are only twenty different kinds of amino acids, but these chemicals can be strung together to make millions of different kinds of substances.

Unlike the vitamins, most of which we have to consume in our diet and supplements since our bodies can't make them, the human body can manufacture all but eight of the amino acids. Those eight amino acids that we need to eat are called *essential* amino acids. The amino acids that can be synthesized from other substances are called *nonessential*.

All Protein Starts in Plants

The protein factories that keep all life on earth supplied with amino acids are plants. These are the only living things that can take inorganic raw materials from the air, soil, and water and, with the help of solar energy, put them together to make protein. All animals either get the organic material to make their proteins from plants or from other animals. Even when our bodies make nonessential amino acids, they make them from organic material that originally came from plants.

Though plants are the original source of protein, the protein in vegetarian foods is considered incomplete. No individual vegetarian food contains all of the essential amino acids in the kind of proportion that allows the human body to make the best use of them. That doesn't mean the protein in vegetables is of lower quality than the protein in meats (which contain complete proteins), it means that you have to eat a variety of vegetarian foods to get complete protein. To get the most vitamins, minerals, and other nutrient factors (many of which have not even been scientifically identified) from your food, you should be eating a variety of vegetarian foods anyway.

Eating the proper mix of vegetarian foods to get complete protein is really a cinch, because complementary proteins—protein foods that together supply all the essential amino acids—are natural match-ups that you probably eat together already, without thinking about their protein content. For instance, if you eat a complete animal protein such as skim milk or cheese with a cereal or grain, you have formed a meal that supplies the proper proportion of amino acids. Cereal with milk, pasta with cheese, and melted cheese on toast all contain complete protein. In addition, peanut butter on bread, rice and beans, or tofu and rice all contain complete protein.

Why is this important to know? Can't you take vitamin supplements and have your burger, too?

Not if you want optimal health. If you take vitamins such as C, E, and beta-carotene because of their possible cardiovascular and anticancer benefits, but you still indulge in large meals of red meat, you are engaging in a nutritional tug of war with yourself. The vitamins may pull in one direction and help you stay healthy, but they will be of reduced value since the diet you are eating is associated with an increased risk of certain cancers and heart disease and is pulling in the opposite direction.

Unknown Factors in Food

When you consume a mostly vegetarian diet along with your vitamin supplement program, you are ingesting many health-promoting factors in food that are poorly understood and are not available in pill form.

For instance, while beta-carotene has intrigued scientists with its antioxidant and antidisease abilities, this chemical is merely one member of the family of substances known as carotenoids that are present in plants and vegetarian foods. The carotenoids are the pigments that give fruits and vegetables their characteristic colors of yellow, red, and orange. Plants do not only make carotenoids for color, it is for their own antioxidant protection, preserving the integrity of plant cells and warding off attacks by free radicals.

Aside from acting as an antioxidant in the human body, beta-carotene can also be made into vitamin A when the necessity arises. Although beta-carotene is the most useful carotenoid for making vitamin A, it is not the only carotenoid that serves this purpose. Thirty-six other carotenoids also can be made into vitamin A. For instance, the carotenoids known as alpha-carotene and delta-carotene also yield vitamin A, albeit much less efficiently. As for most of the other hundreds of carotenes, no one is really sure how efficiently many of them are converted into vitamin A.

One thing that is certain: the carotenes in vegetarian foods travel in groups. You rarely eat a single carotenoid as you do in a beta-carotene supplement. It is possible that the groups of carotenoids convey health benefits that are not available when you merely take that supplement.

Incomplete Knowledge of Carotenoids

A hindrance to the complete understanding of how carotenoids affect our health is the difficulty in making comparisons between how animals in the lab react to nutrients in their diet and how the human body makes use of these substances.

In testing the effects of carotenoids on laboratory

animals such as rats and guinea pigs, scientists have found that few animals can take in and metabolize the wide spectrum of carotenoids that humans are able to utilize. Unless they are fed tremendous amounts of carotenoids, mice and rats, for instance, rarely absorb intact carotenoids the way we do. Other types of animals only absorb certain kinds of carotenoids. For instance, cows take in beta-carotene from grass, which gives butter its characteristic yellow color. In the winter, when cows eat less grass, butter is usually white, but food companies color it with beta-carotene to keep it yellow and keep consumers happy. Chickens absorb carotenoids known as hydroxy carotenoids, which can give some chicken its characteristic yellow coloring.

Because there are few good animal models for the physiological actions of carotenoids, miraculous nutrients could be hiding in this group of substances and no one would know it. What is known about this group of nutrients clearly shows that if you take beta-carotene to improve your health but ignore the importance of a mostly vegetarian diet to round out your health program, you are missing out on some important nutritional benefits.

Just the fact that carotenoids are always found in groups in vegetables suggests that it is important to ingest a variety of these substances rather than relying on a single nutrient. It has been shown that carotenoids interact: A carotenoid called lycopene, for instance, the pigment that gives tomatoes their red color, helps the human body absorb beta-carotene. If you eat a slice of tomato along with your beta-carotene supplement, it will help you take in more of this nutrient.

The fat you eat will also help you absorb beta-carotene, just as fat aids the absorption of vitamins E, D, and K. At the same time, another way to increase your carotene absorption from foods such as carrots is to cook them for a brief period of time.

Studies show that shorter cooking times dramatically increase the amount of beta-carotene absorbed by the digestive system. Cooking vegetables until they are soggy destroys carotenoids, as does boiling. Boiling vegetables also drains off much of their B vitamins. It's best to steam your vegetables or microwave them for a very short time, stopping when they are hot but still crisp. That kind of cooking will maximize your vegetable nutrient intake.

Nutrients Interact With Beta-Carotene

As I've noted previously, nutrition scientists used to think that beta-carotene's main function was to act as a vitamin A precursor—that our bodies only used beta-carotene to make vitamin A when our diets didn't supply enough vitamin A. Now, of course, we know that our bodies absorb intact beta-carotene as ammunition against free radicals that may cause cancer and heart disease (see pages 118–123). Now, in a surprising scientific turnaround, it is being shown that getting enough vitamin A may help us absorb and use more beta-carotene.

In other words, when you take in enough vitamin A, less beta-carotene is converted to vitamin A and more of this nutrient is available in the cells to exercise its antioxidant muscle. Other experiments also show that getting enough protein, zinc, and vitamin E may also help your body use larger amounts of beta-carotene. In ways that scientists don't completely comprehend, all of these nutrients interact within the body. If your diet is seriously deficient in any one of them, the metabolism of the others may become deficient and can help compromise your health.

You can disrupt your beta-carotene absorption by drinking large amounts of alcoholic beverages. Aside from the fact that combining large amounts of beta-carotene with alcohol may damage your liver (see page 119), alcohol limits your liver's ability to store vitamin A and interferes with the liver's conversion of beta-carotene into forms that can be transported in the blood.

Vitamins, Diet, and Lifestyle

When Mr. and Mrs. Average American and their offspring sit down in front of their television set with beer, soda, and potato chips night after night, they are indulging in unhealthy lifestyle practices that no amount of vitamin supplements can possibly offset. Aside from the mental effects of the mind-numbing content of the shows they choose to watch and the lack of exercise this kind of recreation represents, their dietary choices are lacking in essential vitamins, fiber, and minerals that would, in the long run, boost their health.

Most dietitians will tell you that there are no bad or unhealthy foods, there are only poor diets. You may hear that any food, no matter how greasy, fatty, and without apparent redeeming nutritional value, can be eaten in moderation as long as the rest of the diet contains large amounts of fresh fruits and vegetables.

Common sense, however, suggests that this perspective is distorted. How many people down soda, beer, and pretzels as hors d'oeuvres and then have healthy helpings of green salad, legumes, and steamed vegetables? Fast food and sugary drinks merely increase your taste for more of the same.

Statistics that measure our food intake bear this out. The latest figures show that many of us eat hardly any fruits and vegetables at all, that we overindulge in fast food, and when we do eat salads and vegetables, we choose items that don't supply very much of the carotenes, vitamin C, fiber, and other vitamins and fiber.

All this makes for a rather peculiar vitamin status. As we mentioned before, some nutritionists believe that without French fries, scurvy, the vitamin C deficiency disease, would be rampant in the United States, even though potatoes are a relatively poor source of vitamin C. The average American consumes little produce rich in vitamin C, but eats between 70 and 80 pounds of potatoes a year, making this food our second most significant dietary source of vitamin C. Only oranges and orange juice supply more. In third place, as a source of vitamin C for Americans are tomatoes, which are also not superbly rich in vitamin C. We each pack away more than 25 pounds of tomatoes a year, which includes the tomatoes that go into the tomato sauce on everyone's spaghetti, ketchup for the fries, as well as the slices of tomato on BLTs.

The situation is similar though not identical to our dietary sources of beta-carotene. Tomatoes are not a very rich source of beta-carotene, but they are our third highest source of this nutrient because we eat so many of them. Carrots and sweet potatoes are our two main sources for beta-carotene, even though we only average about 9 1/2 pounds of carrots a year and 4 1/2 pounds of sweet potatoes. Since these two vegetables are such rich sources of beta-carotene, these small amounts make a significant impact on our diets.

Also in the top twenty contributors of beta-carotene to our diets are apples, bananas, and oranges, again, not because they are rich sources, but because we eat so much of them.

The nutritional lesson that America's diet teaches is that the typical snacks lack enough beta-carotene and vitamin C, and supplements won't be able to make up the difference. They may slightly improve your nutrition status, but they can't fill in all the gaps left by fat-filled munchies. Supplements represent only a few of the factors in food that you need for good health. These factors may be important, but it isn't even certain that there aren't other factors that may be even more important.

Some of the more nutritious foods that should be the centerpiece of a vegetarian diet would include the legumes (lentils, beans, and peas), peppers, carrots, sweet potatoes, snap beans, lima beans, and winter squash. At the present time, these foods make up a rather minimal part of the American diet. We should eat more of these types of vegetarian foods instead of filling up on meat, iceberg lettuce, tomatoes, and the ubiquitous fried potato.

16

Protein Supplements and Smart Drugs: Boon or Fraud

Protein supplements have been sold for as long as men have taken off their shirts at the beach and displayed their muscles for the benefit of their girlfriends and boyfriends. Of course, nowadays, many women are taking off their shirts and displaying inflated triceps, biceps, and abs as well.

Because of our obsession with the fitness of our bodies and brains, ambitious businesspeople have marketed a bewildering collection of protein powders, pills, and liquids supposedly designed to do everything from making our muscles bulge to evaporating body fat to sharpening our brains. These promises, like many other promises of happiness in a jar, are spurious, and the substances, when taken in large amounts, can be dangerous. In some instances they may even be dangerous in small amounts. Just because vitamins come in pill form and may be beneficial to your health, you should not jump to the conclusion that you can take amino acids and protein the same way.

You need to consume protein every day to repair and rebuild your body because protein isn't stored the way fat and carbohydrates are stored. When you take large amounts in supplement form, however, the excess is merely flushed out of your system; it does not flow to your muscles. Removing this excess protein is not a simple matter for the kidneys and liver. The process gives these organs a lot of extra work as they break down the unneeded amino acids, mix them with water, and pass them out in your urine. If you are prone to any kind of kidney problems, the strain of dealing with the amino acids in protein supplements may instigate kidney failure. Since the body's elimination of amino acids requires a large quantity of water, consuming excess protein can make you dehydrated.

High levels of protein supplementation that is eliminated in your urine can also leach calcium out of your body. Depending on how strong your bones are, over an extended period of time that removal of calcium could make you vulnerable to osteoporosis, an especially serious problem for women whose bone mass is usually lower than men's.

Exaggerated Benefits

In exchange for these potential problems, there are not many proven benefits of protein supplements. For one thing, the proteins in these powders and pills are usually derived from foods you could simply eat at much less cost. A close inspection of ingredient lists shows that the protein is usually taken from soy beans or milk. In many cases, a plate of tofu (made from soy) or a glass of skim milk will supply the same protein that is contained in supplements.

Despite the claims made in ads for predigested protein supplements, the protein on your dinner plate is just as bioavailable as the protein in powders and pills. You can absorb it just as readily. The processing that goes into making protein supplements does not significantly speed or ease the protein's passage through your digestive tract.

Some marketers of protein supplements say that these substances can help you lose weight. That, of course, is nonsense. No scientific evidence has ever been gathered that substantiates this kind of benefit. In particular, arginine and ornithine have been sold as hormone stimulants that will cause your body to speed its metabolism and burn away extra fat, but the amount of amino acids in these supplements is too small to have any such effect. If you did take enough to speed up your metabolism, these amino acids would probably make you dreadfully ill.

Supposed Appetite Suppressant

Another amino acid, phenylalanine, has been marketed as both an appetite suppressant and as an intelligence enhancer. Part of the rationale for claiming this amino acid is beneficial is the fact that the body converts it into norepinephrine, a neurochemical that plays a part in keeping you alert as well as regulating hunger. Contrary to claims by supplement companies, downing phenylalanine pills, powders, or drinks will not stimulate extra production of norepinephrine. The body regulates its production of its neurochemicals through other means, not because of anything you eat.

Consuming quantities of phenylalanine can have other, undesirable consequences. In some people, this amino acid causes irritability and insomnia. In others, those born with a metabolic defect called phenylketonuria (PKU), consuming this substance can cause damage to the nervous system.

People with PKU—1 person in about 15,000—lack an enzyme necessary to break down phenylalanine. When this amino acid builds up in the blood, the nervous system is damaged. Besides being at serious risk from phenylalanine, those with PKU must avoid artificially sweetened foods containing aspartame (also known by its brand name, NutraSweet), which contains the amino acids phenylalanine and aspartic acid.

Protein as a Somnorific

Other claims for amino acid supplements claim that they can both help you sleep better and recover from athletic injury or fatigue faster. Both of these claims are distortions. For one thing, while your recovery from the rigors of exercise may partly depend on the protein you consume, a normal diet contains sufficient amounts of protein for almost any muscle building demands. Protein supplements will not significantly affect this process. When added to the large amount of protein most of us already eat in our diets, these extra amino acids will merely be excreted or burned for energy. Chances are, they'll merely add to the burden of your kidneys and liver when they are eliminated from the body.

As for helping you sleep, a few companies used to market the amino acid tryptophan as a sleep aid since studies had shown that it soothed some insomnia sufferers. However, as noted on page 67, people have died from taking tryptophan supplements and, to date, no one has ever satisfactorily explained what it was in the supplements that killed them.

At the time of the tryptophan deaths, the Food and Drug Administration found that tryptophan takers were falling ill with eosinophilia, an extremely serious blood disease whose symptoms include extreme weakness, fever, rashes, and muscle pains. The source of the disease may have been a contaminant that was inadvertently added to the supplements, which were mostly produced in Japan, or taking tryptophan itself may have caused the condition. In any case, these supplements have been banned in the United States and should not be taken. If you have a jar of these supplements, throw them out or return them to the store where you bought them.

Avoid Amino Acid Supplements

Because of all the medical difficulties associated with amino acid supplements, the Federation of American Societies for Experimental Biology warns that anyone taking these substances puts him/herself at risk. The possible adverse effects mean that these supplements should only be taken while under close medical supervision.

In addition, experts warn that children and pregnant women are at special risk from many of these substances: Supplements containing L-cysteine can harm the fetus of a pregnant woman. Another amino acid found in supplements, taurine, can cause serious reactions in PKU sufferers, as well as in those with Wilson's disease (an inability to properly metabolize copper). Persons taking antidepressant drugs containing chemicals called MAO (monoamine oxidase) inhibitors may be harmed by these supplements, too. These antidepressants include Eutonyl, Parnate, Marplan, and Nardil.

Should You Take Smart Drugs With Your Vitamins?

Many people believe that if establishment scientists fail to recognize all the benefits of vitamin supplements, that it is possible they are also neglecting the benefits of a new class of drugs that have been called smart drugs.

These drugs are prescription items that have been used to treat conditions associated with mental disorders.

Along with their vitamins in the morning, many young professionals, looking for that extra mental and physical edge that will help them succeed in the business world, are taking drugs like Dilantin (phenytoin), Hydergine (ergoloid mesylates), Diapid (phenytoin), and Elepryl (selegiline hydrochloride). These drugs are commonly prescribed to treat diseases such as Parkinson's.

Besides these drugs, according to *FDA Consumer Magazine,* other smart drugs not approved for any use in the United States, but which are being smuggled into the country, include Oxicebral (vincamine), Attentil (fipexide), Nootropil (piracetam), Draganon (aniracetam), and Cavinton (vinpocetine).

The Food and Drug Administration has not approved any of these drugs (or any drugs for that matter) for use in improving intelligence, memory, or business acumen. That fact, of course, does not deter many from using these chemicals in an attempt to boost their mental powers. The alleged scientific rationale behind their usefulness is that since these chemicals are supposed to be effective in the treatment of mental disorders, then they must be able to enhance the mental abilities of those who do not suffer from mind-affecting diseases.

There's no scientific proof that they do anything of the sort. Besides that, there's also little knowledge of what long-term effects and possible dangers might result from taking these drugs.

While laboratory studies have shown that animals learn mazes faster while taking some of these drugs, no proof exists that they will help you do your taxes faster, close more real estate deals, or make a fortune on the stock market. According to Dr. Thomas Crook, who performs research for the Memory Assessment Clinics, Inc., of Bethesda, Maryland, no well constructed study has ever shown that taking these drugs for months or years will improve mental performance in humans.

In an interview with *FDA Consumer*, Dr. Crook, who ran the National Institute of Mental Health's geriatric psychopharmacology program for more than ten years, pointed out that you can't apply the results of studies on animal intelligence to humans.

Although the long-term effects of these drugs are not well understood, the short-term discomforts they can cause are well documented. Diapid can make your nose run, form ulcers in your nasal passages, annoy you with an increase in bowel movements, and cramp your stomach. The unpleasant side effects of Hydergine and Nootropil include nausea, sleep disturbances, headaches, and upset stomach.

Aside from the problems of side effects associated with individual drugs, another danger is the synergistic effects these drugs may produce when taken together. Many believers in the power of these chemicals take cocktails of several of them together. No one knows what this will mean for their health after several years of self-medication.

Black Market Chemicals

According to *FDA Consumer,* marketing and selling these drugs as mind enhancers is illegal in the United States. Importing small amounts (a three-month supply) of these drugs for personal use is permitted by the FDA, but you are not allowed to bring them into the country in large quantities and sell them. However, the FDA believes that black marketers are importing these drugs under the personal-use provisions of the importing laws and then selling them illegally.

Unlike the laws regulating these drugs, there are no laws outlawing amino acid supplements or protein drinks as long as these foodstuffs are not advertised as having health benefits. The FDA is currently pondering new and improved ways to regulate these supplements.

Although many who consider themselves among the hip elite continue to take chemicals supposed to give them super mental powers, it is a risky business. It's better to stick to vitamins whose safety and health benefits are well established.

GLOSSARY

absorption The process in the digestive tract during which vitamins and other nutrients are transported through the epithelial tissue that lines the stomach and intestines and then distributed to the body via the blood or lymph.

acetate This chemical is combined with vitamin A in many vitamin preparations. It is preferable to take your vitamin A as beta-carotene rather than vitamin A acetate.

actinic keratosis A precancerous skin growth that can turn malignant. Often caused by too much time in the sun or under ultraviolet tanning lights, this growth is usually found on the skin of the middle-aged or elderly.

aerobic Using oxygen. Usually refers to aerobic exercise, exercise performed slowly enough so that demand for oxygen does not exceed supply. While aerobic exercise strengthens the cardiovascular system, aerobic production of energy in the cells liberates destructive free radicals, which can cause cellular damage. Antioxidant vitamins along with antioxidants produced by the body can limit this damage.

amino acids The building blocks that make up all

proteins. About twenty make up the proteins in your body. Of these, eight are considered essential amino acids; they have to be eaten in your diet and cannot be synthesized from other compounds. It is not recommended that you take amino acid supplements. Such supplements can cause health problems.

anaerobic Processes that take place in the absence of oxygen. Also refers to microorganisms that are destroyed by oxygen.

antioxidant A vitamin, chemical, enzyme, drug, or other substance that prevents oxidation (the destruction or degradation of cell membranes or other matter by reactive oxygen or free radicals). The antioxidant vitamins include vitamins E and C and the carotenoids. It is believed that beta-carotene is the most biologically active carotenoid that takes part in antioxidant activities. Often the antioxidant vitamins work together to prevent oxidative destruction in the body.

arginine An amino acid sold as a supplement that reputedly aids in weight loss because, together with the amino acid ornithine, it stimulates the release of growth hormone. Its effectiveness as a diet aid is unproven and experts are concerned about other unknown side effects. It is not recommended.

ariboflavinosis A deficiency of riboflavin (vitamin B_2) characterized by tissue inflammation and wounds that take long to heal. Lips become swollen and cracked in the corners, and the eyes may burn and itch.

ascorbic acid The chemical name for vitamin C.

atrophic gastritis An inflammation of the stomach characterized by destruction of the lining of the stomach. This chronic condition is believed by researchers to be a preliminary step in the development of cancer.

beriberi   A deficiency disease caused by the lack of thiamine. This illness attacks the nervous system and is characterized by pain, paralysis, and edema.

beta-carotene   The most biologically active carotenoid. This nutrient is a vitamin A precursor and can be converted to vitamin A by intestinal enzymes as needed by the body. It also functions as an antioxidant without being changed to vitamin A. Orange and yellow fruits and dark green leafy vegetables such as carrots, broccoli, spinach, apricots, squash, and pumpkin contain large amounts of beta-carotene.

bioavailability   A measure of how absorbable and therefore usable certain nutrients are in the body. For example, the iron in meats is more efficiently absorbed than iron in vegetarian sources, so it is said to be more bioavailable.

bioflavonoids   Naturally occuring chemicals that often accompany vitamin C in food. Sometimes called vitamin P, these chemicals are said to aid in the absorption and use of vitamin C in the body, although this has never been proven.

biological activity   How well utilized a particular vitamin is when it is in the body.

caffeine   A drug that stimulates the central nervous system. Caffeine is present in coffee and many soft drinks. Its health effects are controversial. Some experts link this food additive to heart disease and cancer. However, these associations have never been proven and at least one study has shown that drinkers of decaffeinated coffee may suffer more heart disease than regular coffee drinkers.

carcinogen   A chemical or substance that causes cancer.

carcinogenesis The development of cancer.

carcinoma A cancerous tumor that occurs in epithelial tissue.

carnitine A nutrient produced in the body that also occurs in many different foods. Sold as a supplement, carnitine is used in moving fat within each cell of your body so it can be metabolized. There is no generally accepted benefit to taking carnitine supplements.

carotenoids Plant pigments that give fruits, vegetables, and flowers their orange, red, and yellow colors. The green color of chlorophyll in the plant may hide the carotenoid color. There are over 500 carotenoids known to science. Every year, plants produce over 100 million tons of these chemicals. Carotenoids protect plants from the corrosive, oxidative by-products of photosynthesis. When eaten, your body may convert some carotenoids to vitamin A or use them as antioxidants.

chelation The process that binds minerals to amino acids. Supplements of chelated minerals are supposed to be absorbed more efficiently in the digestive tract. However, it is believed that chelation has no effect on vitamin absorption.

cobalamin Chemical name for vitamin B_{12}.

coenzyme A substance that helps an enzyme perform its function in the body. Most vitamins perform coenzyme functions in your body, aiding in the metabolism of nutrients, building cell structures, or aiding in the immune system's battle against disease.

collagen Connective tissue that holds the body together. One of vitamin C's most important functions is taking part in the production of collagen.

cytotoxic testing Blood test designed to show food

allergies. The FDA and other experts do not consider this test a reliable indication of allergies.

disintegration time   The amount of time it takes a vitamin pill, mineral tablet, capsule, or other supplement to break up when tested in the laboratory under conditions similar to that in your digestive tract.

dissolution time   The amount of time it takes a vitamin pill, mineral tablet, capsule, or other supplement to dissolve in chemicals similar to those in your digestive tract. Dissolution time is longer than that for disintegration.

diverticulitis   Inflammation of the intestinal tract characterized by the formation of pouches that can become inflamed and infected. This condition is thought to be related to a low-fiber diet, constipation, and straining to pass small, hard stools. It is often treated with a high-fiber diet. If you think you suffer from this condition, consult your doctor.

DNA (deoxyribonucleic acid)   The genetic material in the cell nucleus that controls cell division and other cellular functions. It is thought that oxidative damage to DNA can cause cancer and aging. Antioxidant vitamins may help prevent this damage.

dysplasia   An abnormal change in the organization, size, and shape of cells in any part of the body that may signal the danger that cancer may develop. Dysplasia is usually considered a premalignant condition.

edema   Swelling, usually of arms or legs, caused by the buildup of liquid in intercellular spaces.

eicosapentanoic acid (EPA)   A type of omega 3 fatty acid, generally found in cold-water fish, that is marketed as a fish oil supplement. This type of fat is supposed to protect against heart disease.

empty calories   Refers to refined foods (donuts, cake, potato chips, etc.) that contain high amounts of sugar and fat and sometimes salt, but few vitamins, minerals, and other nutrients or fiber.

enzymes   Catalysts that speed up processes in the body without undergoing chemical changes in themselves. Usually made of protein, there are believed to be more than 50,000 enzymes in the human body. Many vitamins act as coenzymes, helping enzymes perform their metabolic tasks.

epithelial tissue   The cells that line the surfaces of the body's cavities, including the digestive tract.

epidemiological research (epidemiology)   Studies that examine the development of certain diseases in large populations (often entire countries) and by analyzing the influence of diet, pollution, lifestyle factors, environmental factors, or genetic influences in those populations, tries to discern meaningful patterns and associations among these factors that determine the populations' health status.

ergogenic   Nutrient, vitamin, or food alleged to increase athletic ability.

essential amino acids   Amino acids that you must consume in your diet, which your body cannot synthesize from other dietary components. Individual vegetarian foods do not contain all the essential amino acids in the proper proportions but must be combined to supply complete protein.

essential fatty acids   Fats that your body cannot make, which must be supplied by your diet.

fatty acids The basic materials that make up fat. Fatty acids are necessary for the absorption and use of the fat-soluble vitamins A, D, E, and K.

fiber The indigestible part of vegetarian foods. There are two types of fiber, soluble and insoluble. Soluble fiber, found in oats, beans, and carrots, lowers cholesterol. Insoluble fiber, found in bran and whole grains, may help prevent colon cancer. Because of the wide variety of fibers in food, fiber supplements are not recommended. You should eat a diet fairly high in fiber.

folate (folic acid) B vitamin shown to be instrumental in preventing birth defects resulting from failure of the fetus's neural tube to close.

free radicals Caustic substances in the body that, unchecked, damage cell structures via oxidation. Normal metabolic processes release free radicals as do air pollutants such as cigarette smoke. Free radicals are believed to have a role in causing heart disease, cancer, and other diseases.

glossitis Symptom of riboflavin deficiency characterized by a swollen, dark red tongue.

glycogen The reserve of starch saved by the body that can be used for energy as necessary.

international unit (IU) Measurement unit used to indicate the amounts of vitamins A and E in vitamin supplements.

lactoflavin The name for the chemical form of riboflavin contained in milk.

lecithin A fatlike substance found in egg yolk and

other foods that plays a role in the metabolism of fat. Sold as a supplement, most nutrition experts do not recognize any health benefits attributable to taking lecithin.

lymph The liquid that flows through the lymphatic vessels. The cells in this liquid are immune cells known as lymphocytes. Created in the lymph nodes, lymphocytes battle infectious agents and disease-causing microbes.

metabolism All of the internal chemical processes that keep your body alive and that result in the maintenance and growth of the body's cells, liberation of energy from food, and other chemical changes necessary for health.

metastasis In cancer, this term refers to the spread of the disease from the initial site to a distant organ.

natural Generally refers to vitamins that are derived from organic sources instead of created from scratch in the lab. Some experts recommend taking natural vitamin E (denoted d-alpha-tocopherol), because it is more biologically active than synthetic vitamin E (dl-alpha-tocopherol). It is believed that other vitamins are utilized equally well whether taken in synthetic or natural form. In any case, if everyone who took vitamin C decided to take natural vitamin C instead of the synthetic form, there would not be enough plant life on earth to meet the demand.

neural tube defect A very serious birth defect that occurs when the tube containing nerve tissue that forms the spine and brain does not close properly before birth. This condition has been linked to a folate deficiency in pregnant women.

niacin Vitamin B$_3$.

night blindness Symptom of vitamin A deficiency characterized by the eye's inability to adjust to diminished light.

nitrates Chemicals containing nitrogen that are found in vegetables and soil. Often found as a pollutant in drinking water. When you consume nitrates, they may be changed in the stomach to carcinogenic substances called nitrosamines. Antioxidant vitamins may prevent this conversion.

nitrites Chemicals containing nitrogen that are used to preserve smoked meats and cheese. Also found in beer. When you consume nitrites, they may be changed in the stomach to carcinogenic substances called nitrosamines. Antioxidant vitamins may prevent this conversion.

nitrosamines Carcinogens formed in the stomach from nitrites and nitrates. Antioxidant vitamins may prevent this conversion.

omega 3 fatty acids A type of polyunsaturated fat found in fish and cold water animals (such as seals). The consumption of these nutrients in fish is credited with protecting Eskimos from heart disease. Eicosaspentanoic acid (EPA) is a type of omega 3 fatty acid that is marketed as a fish oil supplement.

ornithine An amino acid sold as a supplement that reputedly aids in weight loss because, together with the amino acid arginine, it stimulates the release of growth hormone. Its effectiveness as a diet aid is unproven and experts are concerned about other unknown side effects. It is not recommended.

osteomalacia Weakening of the bones that usually

results from deficiency of calcium and/or vitamin D.

osteoporosis Weakening of the bones resulting from loss of calcium. This condition occurs most often in older women and is thought to be related to postmenopausal hormonal changes, lack of weight-bearing exercise, and calcium deficiencies. Heredity also plays a part. Methods for prevention are still controversial.

oxidation The destruction or deterioration of a substance by reacting with oxygen or other oxidative agents such as free radicals. Outside the body, the rusting of metals, fats turning rancid, and the disintegration of rubber are examples of oxidation. In the body, oxidation may take place when free radical by-products of metabolism or pollutants from cigarette smoke or smog react with cell membranes and other cell structures.

palmitate A type of fatty acid linked to vitamin A when vitamin A is added to many foods. Palmitate is also combined with vitamin A in many vitamin preparations. In vitamin pills, it is preferable to take your vitamin A as beta-carotene rather than vitamin A palmitate.

pangamic acid Sometimes referred to as vitamin B_{15}, this controversial substance is reputed to aid athletic performance. However, there is no universally accepted definition of pangamic acid's ingredients. The most commonly accepted is a mixture of calcium gluconate and dimethylglycine. Reliable research has not indicated any health or athletic benefit for pangamic acid supplementation.

pellagra Deficiency disease caused by the lack of niacin. It is characterized by diarrhea, skin rashes, and mental disturbances.

pantothenic acid   One of the B vitamins that is generally in plentiful supply in most people's diets.

pernicious anemia   A blood disorder caused by lack of vitamin B_{12} in the diet or an inability to utilize vitamin B_{12}. It most often strikes Caucasians over forty years old and frequently must be treated with injections of vitamin B_{12}.

placebo   A sugar pill or other substance that has no significant biological activity. In double-blind tests, placebos are given to control groups to determine if the substance being tested (and given to another group) has any statistically significant effect on subjects. Placebos are made to taste and appear identical to the drug or vitamin being tested.

placebo effect   Refers to the fact that placebos often seem to make subjects feel better and produce other positive effects even though the substance in the placebo pill is merely sugar or some other inert ingredient that should have no biological effect.

precursor   A substance that the body can convert into another chemical. For example, beta-carotene is often considered a precursor of vitamin A because the body can convert it to vitamin A as needed. While this conversion used to be considered beta-carotene's primary function, it is now known that even without being changed to vitamin A, beta-carotene fulfills an important role as an antioxidant.

prostaglandins   Chemicals (long-chain fatty acids) produced by the body that affect certain processes such as blood clotting and inflammation. It is thought that aspirin prevents pain and restricts blood clotting by its effect on the action of prostaglandins.

provitamin A nutrient that can be converted into a vitamin (see *precursor*).

pyridoxine The chemical name for vitamin B_6.

RDA (recommended dietary allowance) The amounts of vitamins, minerals, and other nutrients consumed daily that are supposed to be adequate for maintaining good health. Arrived at by a committee called the Food and Nutrition Board of the National Research Council, these values are broken down by sex and age and also include values for pregnant and nursing women. Many experts believe the allowances are too low to produce optimal health and are too focused on merely preventing overt deficiencies. These values were originally devised for use by nutrition professionals. USRDAs, more generalized values of vitamins and other nutrients, were designed to be used on food and supplement labels for public information.

RDI (recommended daily intake) The amounts of vitamins, minerals, and other nutrients that are supposed to be adequate to support minimal health standards for the average person. These measurements, designed to be used on food and vitamin labels, are generally lower than the USRDAs that they are designed to replace.

retinol The form of vitamin A that is contained in egg yolks, whole milk, butter, liver, and fish oils.

retinol equivalent (RE) The most recently adapted measurement of vitamin A content, although most vitamin bottles still use the older standard, international units, to report how much vitamin A is in supplements. Each retinol equivalent equals 3.3 international units.

riboflavin Vitamin B_2.

scurvy   A deficiency disease caused by the lack of vitamin C in the diet. This condition is characterized by bleeding gums, easy bruising, joint pain, poor wound healing, and loose teeth.

spina bifida   A birth defect resulting when the fetal neural tube fails to close. This condition is often linked to a folate deficiency in pregnant women.

superoxide dismutase (SOD)   An antioxidant chemical produced in the body that protects cell structures from free radical damage. Sold as a supplement, it is not considered effective. When you swallow this nutrient, it is broken down in the digestive tract into its component protein and is not absorbed intact. It is not recommended.

thiamine   Vitamin B1.

tannins   Chemicals in coffee and tea that diminish your body's absorption of dietary iron.

tryptophan   An amino acid once sold as a supplement, now banned by the FDA because of safety questions. In the body, tryptophan is converted into niacin. You should never take tryptophan supplements. They can be extremely deleterious to your health.

USRDA   (United States recommended daily allowance) A general measurement of vitamins and other nutrients reflecting the amount the average American should be taking in every day. These numbers are designed for use on food and vitamin labels. The FDA wants to replace these numbers with RDIs (recommended daily intakes), which would have lower values.

Wilsons disease   A hereditary inability to properly metabolize copper in the diet. In this condition, copper builds up on the brain and other organs, causing serious damage.

KEEP TRACK OF YOUR DIET
—AND YOUR HEALTH!